CONTENTS

DEDICATION

This book is dedicated to our children who light up our lives—Adam, Anne, Marnie and Hope Frisch, and Jon and Ryan Rapoport—with our wish that everyone will have children to share in the joys of parenthood!

A special thanks to our spouses—Patti Frisch and Jim Rapoport—for their understanding and support.

We would like to pay special tribute to the memory of each of our fathers—Isadore Harold Frisch and Julius Chanen—who gave us the gift of life and the knowledge and encouragement to grow. We miss you both.

Introduction

My interest in pregnancy and infertility dates back to when I first began practicing general medicine in the small, rural communities of Poplar and Wolf Point, Montana in 1967. In those small communities, I realized my patients didn't want to be dictated to by their doctor but were interested in someone who would sit down and explain, in simple terms, what was wrong with them and what could be done.

During the 5 years my wife and I spent in rural Montana, we didn't have a fertility problem—we came childless to Montana in 1967 and left in 1972 with three children, ages 4, 3 and 2. My wife attributed our superfertility to the saddle we had for our horse, Rebel; when she rode the horse, she got pregnant!

We found ourselves too busy with three young children to do much riding, so we loaned our horse and saddle to a friend, who subsequently had two children over the next 2 years. When we left Montana to return to Minnesota for my Obstetrics-Gynecology residency, a going-away party was held for us at the friends' house to whom we had loaned our horse and saddle. The saddle was sitting on a bench in the living room when another couple, who had been trying to conceive for several years, overheard our story about the saddle and subsequent pregnancies. Deciding there was nothing to lose, the infertile woman sat briefly on the saddle to see if it would help her become pregnant. Much to our surprise, about 9 months after our going-away party, we received a birth announcement from our previously infertile friends!

As I worked through my residency, I became very interested in the problems couples have with fertility. When I finished in 1975, I decided to make the study of infertility special in my practice. Today, infertility and tubal microsurgery have become a special interest of mine. But because of the "success" it has brought in the past, it has crossed my mind more than once to bring that saddle out of our basement and place it in the waiting room of my office—perhaps the saddle is one cure for unexplained infertility!

Since completing my residency 11 years ago, I have had a general obstetrical-gynecological practice in the Minneapolis area, with a special interest in infertility. My approach to patients has been the same as it was when I was in Montana—communicating in as simple terms as possible what is wrong with a patient and what can be done for them.

A few years ago, I was approached by my co-author, Gayle Rapoport, to work on a book with her on infertility. She wanted to write a book that people with a non-medical background could understand. One thing led to another, and before I knew it, together we had written this book. It wasn't easy writing a book about such a technical subject in simple terminology, but hopefully we have accomplished our task. This book is not only for couples who have difficulty becoming pregnant but also for any couple planning a pregnancy.

Melvin J. Frisch, M.D.
Minneapolis, 1987

1

What Is Infertility?

Fertility is a personal problem for many people. When a couple has difficulty getting pregnant, we have found it is the woman who *first* starts to believe there might be a fertility problem, and she is the one who begins to seek answers to her questions.

Because we wanted to make this book personal, like a physician talking with a patient, we kept this in mind as we wrote. That's why we wrote it from a woman's point of view—to answer many of the questions you might have when you first suspect there might be a problem with becoming pregnant. We know men are *not* disinterested in infertility and its causes; a man is often just as anxious as his wife about the problems they are having as a couple conceiving a child. But it's the woman's body that first foretells difficulty in conceiving a child—when she doesn't get pregnant!

We hope you will understand and accept the way we have chosen to present our information. We have tried to treat both of you as personally as if you were in the office.

1. *What is infertility?*

Infertility is defined as the inability to become pregnant after trying for 1 year. This assumes regular sexual intercourse has occurred without any form of contraception. There are two types of infertility—primary infertility and secondary infertility. Infertility is also defined as a couple's inability to produce a living child.

2. *What is primary infertility?*

Primary infertility is when a couple has never been able to conceive.

3. *What is secondary infertility?*

Secondary infertility is infertility that occurs after a couple has previously conceived a child.

4. *What are the major causes of infertility?*

Nearly 40% of all infertility problems are attributed to the man; problems include a low sperm count and/or poor motility of sperm.

A woman's failure to ovulate accounts for almost 25% of infertility cases, tubal blockage accounts for about 20%, and a cervical factor, such as poor cervical mucus, is responsible in nearly 5% of the cases.

In about 10% of the couples who experience infertility, no cause can be found.

5. *What is sterility?*

When a man or woman is unable to produce off-spring under any circumstances, he or she is considered sterile and is permanently infertile.

6. *What percentage of all couples are infertile?*

Fifteen percent of all couples are infertile. One in every six couples of childbearing age have a problem conceiving. This amounts to over 10 million people in the United States with a fertility problem.

7. *Is infertility a female condition?*

No. Men, as well as women, can be infertile. In 50% of all couples who are infertile, a female factor is found. A male factor is found in the other 40%. Combined male and female factors are found in 20% of all couples.

8. *What is an example of a combined factor in infertility?*

One example is a man with a borderline sperm count and a woman who is not ovulating. *Both* partners contribute to the infertility.

9. *Is stress a major factor in infertility?*

It is not usually a major factor, but severe stress may contribute to infertility by interfering with your ovulation.

10. *Is infertility a sexual disorder?*

No, it isn't. In most cases, infertility has nothing to do with the ability to perform sexually.

11. *Can infertility be treated?*

Yes, it can. Over 50% of all couples who seek help for their infertility eventually become pregnant. Only 5% who do not seek help become pregnant.

12. *What is the average length of time for a couple to become pregnant?*

Twenty-five percent of all couples become pregnant within the first month of trying. Sixty percent of all couples become pregnant within 6 months, and 85% become pregnant within 1 year. The remaining 15% are considered infertile because they do not achieve pregnancy within 1 year. The average time to achieve pregnancy is 4 to 6 months.

13. *Is infertility on the increase?*

Yes, it appears to be. Researchers believe there are several reasons for this. The first reason is the tendency for couples to delay having children until they are over 30 years old. The second reason is the increase in sexual promiscuity; sexually transmitted diseases can interfere with fertility. The third reason is that past methods of birth control, such as the intrauterine device (IUD), have led to an increase in pelvic infections, which affect fertility.

14. *Does my age affect fertility?*

The prime fertility age in women is the early 20s. Fertility decreases during a woman's 30s, especially after age 35. However, if you are older, it doesn't necessarily mean you will have trouble becoming pregnant. Today, many women delay having their first child until their late 30s and even early 40s.

15. *Does my husband's age affect fertility?*

In men, age usually has no bearing, assuming the semen analysis is normal. Men can remain fertile well into their 60s and even as old as 70 or 80.

16. *Does the miscarriage rate go up as I get older?*

Yes, it does. Miscarriages occur in about 15% of all women between the ages of 30 and 40. In the 35-to-40-year-old age range, the percentage is about 18%. About 25% of the women who become pregnant after age 40 miscarry.

17. *Does my age determine when we should see a doctor?*

If you're under 30, contact a doctor after you have tried to become pregnant for 1 year. If you're over 30, see a doctor after trying to conceive for 6 months. Some women prefer seeing their doctor *before* trying to become pregnant.

18. *What type of doctor should we consult?*

Seek a doctor who is interested in infertility. This is usually an obstetrician-gynecologist (OB-GYN).

19. *When should my husband see a doctor?*

A man usually does not seek primary treatment for infertility until after his wife does. Your doctor will arrange for a semen analysis, and the results of that test will determine whether further testing is necessary for your husband.

20. *What if further testing is necessary?*

If further testing is needed, it's usually done by a urologist who is interested in male infertility.

21. *Do family doctors do infertility testing?*

Many family doctors are capable of evaluating a couple's infertility.

22. *What is an obstetrician?*

An obstetrician is a doctor who cares for a pregnant woman and delivers her baby.

23. *What is a gynecologist?*

A gynecologist is a doctor who takes care of women, with emphasis on their reproductive system. Many gynecologists are also obstetricians.

24. *What is a urologist?*

A urologist is a doctor who specializes in disorders of the urinary system in men and women, and disorders of the male reproductive system.

25. *What is an andrologist?*

An andrologist is a doctor who specializes in the study of sperm production and transport.

26. *What is an endocrinologist?*

An endocrinologist is a doctor who specializes in diseases of the endocrine glands, such as the pituitary, thyroid or adrenal glands.

27. *What is a reproductive endocrinologist?*

A reproductive endocrinologist is a doctor who specializes in the hormones of reproduction. This usually is a gynecologist who has had further training in infertility and the hormones of reproduction.

28. *What is a fertility specialist?*

A fertility specialist is a doctor, such as a gynecologist or urologist, who has a special interest in infertility investigation and treatment.

29. *What special training does a fertility specialist have?*

A doctor who becomes an OB-GYN has a minimum of 4 additional years of training beyond medical school. To become a reproductive endocrinologist requires 2 *more* years of training. Urologists and andrologists have training of similar lengths. Some doctors develop a special interest in infertility and devote most of their practice to it.

30. *How do we choose a doctor?*

One of the best ways to find a doctor is from recommendations of friends or relatives who have been satisfied with their doctor. The local county medical society may also be contacted for referrals.

31. *What if we can't afford a doctor in private practice?*

The county medical association in your area should be able to give you the names of physicians who see patients at reduced rates or for no charge. The name of a free clinic in your area may also be obtained from:
Planned Parenthood Federation of America
810 7th Ave.
New York, NY 10019

32. *What should we look for in a doctor?*

The doctor you choose should be competent, patient, supportive, non-judgmental and inspire confidence in you.

33. *What if we aren't satisfied with our doctor?*

If you feel your doctor is knowledgeable, give him a chance. If you're still dissatisfied, look for another doctor.

34. *Is it common to go from doctor to doctor?*

It is not uncommon to switch doctors; you must do what is best for you. Sometimes a new doctor has a different viewpoint or is more sensitive to your needs. If you change doctors, the new doctor may ask you to repeat some tests that have already been performed.

35. *What if we don't understand what our doctor tells us?*

It's your body, and you have the right to know anything that pertains to you and your care. Don't be afraid to ask questions or to ask your doctor to give you explanations in terms you can understand.

36. *Should we become familiar with medical terminology?*

You're not expected to know medical terminology, but as time goes on, you will probably become familiar with terms that are commonly used. Infertility is not easy to understand in non-medical terms, so it's helpful to try to understand the medical terminology pertaining to your reproductive system.

2

How Do Our Reproductive Systems Work?

The reproductive systems of men and women are extremely complex. Each includes commonly known organs, such as the uterus and ovaries in a woman and the testicles and penis in a man. But less commonly known organs, such as the pituitary and hypothalmus glands (located in the brain), are also part of the reproductive system.

In trying to understand the reasons that contribute to infertility, it helps to know how the reproductive systems work. It's important to understand the chain of events necessary for conception to occur. It also helps you understand why your doctor may perform certain tests.

1. *When does reproduction first become possible for a man or woman?*

The ability to reproduce one's own offspring begins when the sexual organs mature. The age at which this occurs can vary greatly and ranges from age 8 to 18.

Girls usually reach this point about age 12 or 13; boys do not reach this age until about 13 or 14.

2. *What is puberty?*

Puberty is defined as the state of physical development of a child when sexual reproduction first becomes possible; a child starts to mature sexually and sexual organs begin to function. It is a time when a child goes through growth spurts, and there is a rapid increase in height and weight.

3. *What happens to girls during puberty?*

Girls start to develop breasts. This is followed by the appearance of pubic and axillary hair and the beginning of menstruation.

4. *What happens to boys during puberty?*

Boys develop facial and pubic hair, and their testicles and penis increase in size.

5. *At what age does puberty start?*

This varies greatly. A girl usually starts her growth spurt about age 10 to 11, 1 to 2 years earlier than boys. There usually is a 2-year time interval between the first sign of breast development in a girl and the onset of menstruation. The average age for the start of puberty in girls is 10 to 11, with the onset of menstruation at about 12-1/2 years old. The average age for boys to start puberty is age 12 to 13.

6. *What causes puberty?*

The hypothalmus starts to mature and sends out GNRH (gonadotropin-releasing hormone) to the pituitary gland—an endocrine gland located in the brain that secretes hormones that affect body growth and metabolism. The pituitary gland sends out the hormones *FSH* (follicular stimulating hormone) and *LH* (luteinizing hormone) to the ovaries in a woman and the testicles in a man.

In a woman, ovaries are stimulated to produce the hormones estrogen and progesterone, which are responsible for breast development and the onset of menstruation.

In a man, the testicles produce the hormone testosterone, which stimulates the testicles to produce sperm, the penis to grow to adult size and hair to grow on the face.

7. *What is a hormone?*

A hormone is a substance produced by an endocrine gland, such as the ovaries, testicles, thyroid or adrenal gland. The hormone passes into the bloodstream and is carried to other organs or tissues, where it modifies their structure or function. A hormone is like a messenger that tells other organs what to do.

8. *What is an endocrine gland?*

An endocrine gland is an organ that secretes hormones into the blood that influence metabolism and other body processes. Examples of endocrine glands related to reproduction include the ovaries and testicles, and the hypothalmus, pituitary, thyroid and adrenal glands.

9. *What is the hypothalmus?*

It is a region in the brain that slowly matures during childhood; at maturation it causes the reproductive system to develop. The hypothalmus secretes GNRH, which stimulates the pituitary gland to produce its hormones. Without GNRH, the pituitary gland, ovaries and uterus would not work.

10. *Does the hypothalmus have other functions?*

Yes, it does. It's the temperature-regulating area in the brain that causes your body temperature to rise when you are sick. It also has other functions not related to fertility.

11. *How does GNRH affect fertility?*

Under extremely stressful conditions, the hypothalmus can reduce the secretion of GNRH; menstrual cycles may become irregular and even stop.

12. *What is the pituitary gland?*

The pituitary gland is the master gland of the body and is located at the base of the skull, between and behind the eyes. It receives messages from the hypothalmus through GNRH. The pituitary gland sends FSH and LH to the ovaries and testicles so they produce estrogen and progesterone in a woman and testosterone in a man.

13. *Does the pituitary gland produce sex hormones?*

Only indirectly through its effect on the ovaries and testicles. Once the pituitary gland receives GNRH from the hypothalmus gland, it produces FSH and LH, which in turn stimulate the ovaries and testicles to produce "sex" hormones.

14. *How do FSH and LH work in a woman?*

FSH travels through the bloodstream and stimulates the eggs in the ovary to ripen; it gets the ovary ready to ovulate. Then LH takes over and causes the egg to be released from the ovary. This process of developing an egg and expelling it out of the ovary is called *ovulation*.

15. *How do FSH and LH work in a man?*

FSH stimulates the tubules in the testicles to produce sperm. LH stimulates the Leydig cells in the testicles to produce testosterone.

16. *Does the pituitary gland secrete other hormones?*

Yes. In addition to FSH and LH, it produces prolactin, which causes the breasts to secrete milk, thyroid-stimulating hormone (TSH), which regulates the thyroid gland, adrenocorticotropic hormone (ACTH), which controls the adrenal gland, and growth hormone (GH), which controls the way the body grows.

17. *Can abnormalities of the pituitary gland affect fertility?*

Yes, they can. Small growths or tumors in the pituitary gland, called *pituitary adenomas* or *microadenomas,* can cause infertility.

18. *How do these growths cause infertility?*

Even though these tumors may not cause any other symptoms, they can cause an overproduction of hormones from the pituitary gland. This overproduction results in overstimulation of the glands the pituitary affects, such as the thyroid and adrenal glands. Overstimulation results in an excessive amount of thyroid or adrenal hormones, which may affect fertility through its feedback system on the pituitary. Thyroid or adrenal hormones interact with FSH and LH and interfere with ovulation.

19. *How do these hormones interact with each other?*

Most of the pituitary hormones work by a system called the *negative-feedback system.* When more of a pituitary hormone is secreted, such as FSH, it results in more estrogen being produced by the ovaries.

Production of more estrogen causes a *decrease* in FSH production by the pituitary gland. This results in less estrogen production, which results in an *increase* in FSH.

There is a fine balance between the production of

the specific hormone the pituitary gland produces and the hormone produced by the gland it is stimulating. See illustration on opposite page.

20. *What is prolactin, and how can it affect fertility?*

Prolactin is a hormone that appears to play a major part in infertility. It is produced by the pituitary gland, and it stimulates the breasts to produce milk after you have a baby. Under certain conditions, small growths occur in the prolactin-producing cells of the pituitary gland, which result in the production of a large amount of prolactin.

21. *How does a large amount of prolactin affect fertility in a man and in a woman?*

An increase in prolactin causes a suppression of FSH and LH. Prolactin has an inverse relationship with FSH and LH. A decrease in FSH and LH results in less stimulation of the ovaries by FSH and LH, with a possible inhibition of ovulation.

22. *What are the symptoms of an increase in prolactin secretion?*

An increased prolactin secretion may cause you to leak a milky substance from your breast, even in a non-pregnant state. It may also cause your periods to stop.

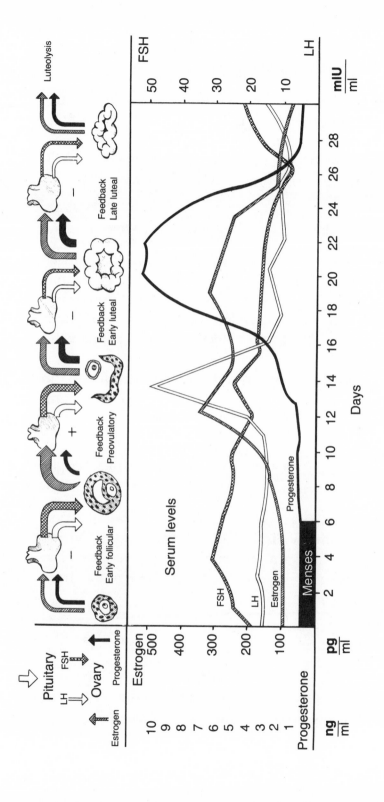

Correlation of serum gonadotropic and ovarian levels and feedback mechanisms.

17

23. *What is this condition called?*

The condition in which a milky substance is discharged from the breast is called *galactorrhea;* the condition in which your periods stop is called *amenorrhea.* When these two conditions appear together, it is called the *amenorrhea-galactorrhea syndrome.*

24. *How does amenorrhea-galactorrhea syndrome occur?*

The production of a large amount of prolactin causes a decrease of FSH and LH. The decrease in FSH and LH results in a decrease in estrogen production by the ovaries, with subsequent lack of estrogen stimulation to the uterine lining and a blockage of ovulation by the ovaries.

Increased prolactin results in stimulation of the breasts to produce milk. There is no uterine lining buildup, no periods and no ovulation.

25. *How can amenorrhea-galactorrhea syndrome be detected?*

Your doctor will ask you if you have irregular periods or any milky discharge from the breasts. During your physical exam, he may gently massage your breasts to see if he can expel milky secretion from either nipple.

26. *What test determines the presence of prolactin?*

If your doctor feels it's necessary, he will order a blood test, called a *serum prolactin,* to determine the amount of prolactin in your bloodstream.

27. *What if the blood test shows I'm producing too much prolactin?*

This may indicate the presence of a tumor, called an *adenoma*. An X-ray or CT scan of the pituitary gland shows if a tumor is present.

28. *What is the treatment for a pituitary adenoma?*

If a large growth is present, surgery may be necessary to remove the tumor. If the tumor is very small, bromocryptine (Parlodel) is used to lower the level of prolactin to normal and shrink the tumor's growth.

29. *Do these methods of treatment cure the infertility problem?*

If this caused your infertility, it should cure the problem.

30. *Are there other causes of an increased prolactin blood test?*

Yes. Certain medications, such as potent tranquilizers (Thorazine, Mellaril) and birth-control pills, can occasionally cause increased prolactin levels. Hypothyroidism may also cause elevated prolactin and galactorrhea.

31. *Are there other symptoms of a pituitary tumor?*

If the tumor is very large, it may cause headaches or vision difficulties. The pituitary gland is located between and behind the eyes, so the enlarged gland may press on nerves that go to the eye. This pressure may produce a visual-field defect, such as loss of part of the visual field. This is the reason your doctor may ask you about headaches and check your vision as part of an infertility examination.

32. *Can men have pituitary tumors?*

Yes. A pituitary tumor in a man can cause a milky secretion from his breasts. If a growth is large enough, it can also cause headaches or vision difficulties.

33. *Can pituitary growths affect a man's fertility?*

Yes. These growths can lower a man's sperm count to a very low level. A growth causes a decrease in FSH stimulation and a decrease in sperm production by the seminiferous tubules. It is advisable to check serum prolactin in any man with a low sperm count.

34. *Are pituitary tumors benign?*

They are in most cases. If they become large, they can be more serious. Rarely, they become malignant and may spread to other parts of the body.

35. *What is the thyroid gland?*

The thyroid gland is a gland located in the neck, in front of the trachea (windpipe). It manufactures the hormone thyroxin, which controls metabolism in the body.

36. *What controls the thyroid gland?*

The thyroid gland is controlled by a hormone from the pituitary gland called thyroid-stimulating hormone (TSH).

37. *Can abnormalities of the thyroid gland cause infertility?*

Yes. Too much or too little thyroid hormone can cause infertility.

38. *How do thyroid abnormalities affect a woman?*

Abnormal levels of thyroid hormone may cause ovulation and menstrual disorders. Your menstrual periods may become irregular or very heavy. It can also cause your periods to stop.

39. *How do thyroid abnormalities affect a man?*

They can interfere with the production of sperm in a man.

40. *How are abnormalities of the thyroid gland detected?*

Several different blood tests can detect abnormalities of the thyroid gland. They include a serum-TSH test, T3 and T4 tests, and a free-thyroxin test. Your doctor will know which test is best for you.

41. *I've heard taking thyroid medication will help fertility, even if a thyroid test is normal. Is this true?*

Years ago, thyroid was given to almost all infertile couples (both men and women), even if thyroid function was normal. There is no evidence this improved fertility.

Some of these couples conceived, but it is believed they would have conceived even without taking the medication. There is no evidence thyroid medication should be given to *anyone* with normal thyroid function for fertility purposes.

42. *What is the adrenal gland?*

The adrenal gland consists of a pair of small endocrine glands—one sits on top of each kidney. Together they produce many different hormones that control various bodily functions.

43. *What are some of the hormones the adrenal gland produces?*

The adrenal gland produces a group of hormones called *glucocorticoids*—cortisol is the most well-known. These hormones control sugar metabolism in the body.

A group of hormones called *mineralcorticoids* are also produced—aldosterone is the most widely known. The main function of mineralcorticoids is control of sodium and potassium metabolism, with subsequent control of blood pressure.

44. *What controls the adrenal gland?*

The adrenal gland is stimulated and controlled by the hormone ACTH (adrenocorticotropic hormone), which is produced by the pituitary gland.

45. *Do the adrenal glands produce sex hormones?*

Yes, they do. The adrenal gland produces androgens (male hormones) and estrogens (female hormones). Both these hormones are produced in men *and* women. Under normal circumstances, androgen and estrogen production by the adrenal gland in a woman is very small compared to the production of these same hormones by the ovaries. Under certain conditions, excessive amounts of these hormones are produced in men and women.

46. *What happens when excessive amounts of adrenal sex hormones are produced?*

In a woman, an excessive amount of adrenal sex hormones results in excessive hair growth, acne and increased muscular development. These hormones may also cause irregular periods and cessation of ovulation. Excessive amounts of adrenal hormones may affect sperm production in a man.

47. *What causes excessive adrenal-hormone production?*

Tumors (benign or malignant) similar to pituitary-gland tumors may cause excessive adrenal-hormone production. A condition called *hyperplasia*, which is an enlarged grouping of cells, can also cause excessive hormone production. Each hyperplastic cell produces a certain amount of hormones, so more hormones are produced by the cells. If this affects the sex-hormone-producing cells, it results in large amounts of sex hormones produced by the adrenal gland.

48. *How are abnormalities of the adrenal gland discovered?*

A general physical exam can indicate abnormalities of the adrenal gland. Your doctor can tell by your blood pressure, how your body fat is distributed, excessive facial hair and acne. He will determine if further testing is necessary.

49. *What tests detect abnormalities of the adrenal gland?*

Blood tests, including plasma-cortisol levels, serum testosterone and serum dehydroepiandosterone sulfate (DHEAS), are used to detect adrenal-gland abnormalities.

50. *Do other tests have to be performed?*

If blood tests are abnormal, X-rays of the kidneys or a CT scan may be necessary to detect abnormal growths of the adrenal gland.

51. *What treatments are available for these hormone abnormalities?*

It depends on what is wrong. If a tumor or growth causes abnormalities, surgery is required. Mild hormone elevations may be controlled with low-dose cortisone, such as prednisone, to suppress ACTH production and lower hormone production by the adrenal gland.

52. *Do these treatments solve infertility problems?*

Treatment results in a return to normal of your menstrual cycle or a return to normal of sperm production in a man if that was the only cause of infertility. This may solve your fertility problem.

53. *How do my hormones relate to fertility?*

For you to become pregnant, ovulation must occur. For ovulation to occur, the hypothalmus, pituitary, thyroid and adrenal glands and the ovaries must all be synchronized with each other. Ovulation and menstruation are the end result of the interaction of the endocrine glands and the hormones they produce. If there is a problem with *any* part of this interaction, pregnancy will not occur. The same is also true for sperm production in a man.

FEMALE GENITAL ORGANS

It's important for you to be familiar with your reproduction system and female organs. The external parts of the female genitals include the labia majora and labia minora (commonly called the *vulva)*, the clitoris, hymen, Bartholin glands and Skene's glands. The internal reproductive organs include the vagina, uterus (including the cervix and the main body of the uterus), Fallopian tubes and ovaries. See illustrations on pages 27 and 28.

54. *What is the vulva?*

The vulva is the external genital area in a woman. It includes the labia majora, labia minora and the mons pubis, which is the area where the pubic hair grows.

55. *What are the labia majora?*

They are the hairy folds of skin on each side of the opening of the vagina. The labia majora are part of the vulva, and they contain sebaceous and sweat glands. The labia majora are often called the *outer lips* of the female genital system.

56. *What are the labia minora?*

They are two thin skin folds that are usually concealed by the labia majora. In some women, these are very large and project beyond the labia majora. The labia minora are often called the *inner lips* of the female genital system.

57. *What is the urethra?*

In a woman, the urethra is a canal about 1-1/2 inches long that runs from the urinary bladder, along the top portion of the vaginal wall, and empties just above the vaginal opening. It is situated between the vaginal opening and the clitoris.

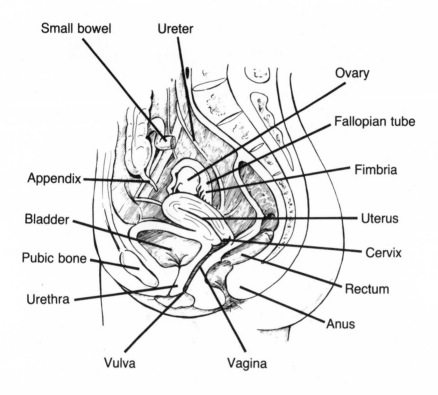

Female pelvic area.

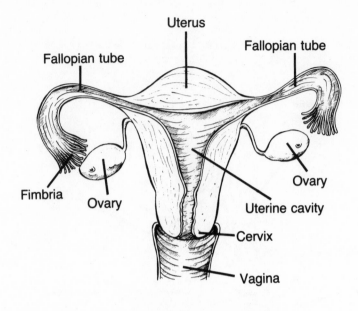

Front view of female reproductive system.

58. *What is the clitoris?*

It is an elongated body of tissue similar to the penis because both are erectile tissue. The clitoris is located at the top of the vulva above the urethral opening, and it acts as a "nerve-center" during intercourse. Sexual stimulation causes veins to fill with blood, which is similar to what occurs in the penis at the time of an erection. When the veins fill with blood, the clitoris becomes elongated and more erect.

59. *What is the hymen?*

The hymen is a membranous fold of vaginal tissue that partially covers the vaginal opening. It is often called the *virginal membrane*. A very tight hymen may prevent the penis from entering the vagina during intercourse. If the hymenal opening cannot be made larger with finger dilatation, tampons or dilators, a *hymenotomy* may be required to make the opening larger.

60. *What is a hymenotomy?*

A hymenotomy is an operation in which small cuts are made in the hymen so the opening is larger. In some cases, part of the hymenal ring may be removed; this is called a *hymenectomy*.

61. *What are the Bartholin glands?*

These glands are located on each side of the vaginal opening in the vulva. They are also called *vulvovaginal glands* and are similar to Cowper's glands in a man because both glands develop from the same tissue. Bartholin glands secrete mucus during sexual stimulation. The opening to these glands may become blocked with retention of its secretions and form a Bartholin duct cyst (a plugged duct).

62. *What are Skene's glands?*

Skene's glands are two small glands located at the base of the urethral opening. They do not have any real function but may become infected if you have a venereal disease. It is believed they are similar to the prostate gland in a man.

63. *What is the vagina?*

The vagina is a tubular structure that extends from the vulva to the cervix. It receives the penis during intercourse, and it is the place where sperm are deposited, leading to conception and pregnancy.

64. *What is the uterus?*

The uterus is a pear-shaped, muscular organ, about 3 inches long. It consists of a flattened part (the body) and a cylindrical part (the cervix or neck). Its cavity opens into the vagina and into the Fallopian tubes on each side. The uterus serves as the incubator and home for a developing fetus.

The lining of the uterus builds up each month under the influence of estrogen and progesterone production from the ovaries and prepares for a developing pregnancy. If pregnancy does not occur, the uterine lining is shed; this is called a *menstrual period*.

65. *What is the cervix?*

The cervix is the lower part of the uterus that protrudes into the top of the vagina. It contains many glands that secrete a watery mucus during the menstrual cycle. The mucus is at its peak in quantity and clarity at ovulation, which enables sperm to easily enter the uterine cavity and progress into the Fallopian tube. The external cervix, called the *exocervix*, is located at the top of the vagina. This is the area that is scraped when a Pap smear is done.

66. *What are Fallopian tubes?*

Each Fallopian tube is a slender tube that extends from the top of the uterus to an ovary. The end of a Fallopian tube, called the *fimbria*, is usually located next to, but not attached to, an ovary.

Normally there are two Fallopian tubes, one on each side of the uterus, that go to the corresponding ovary on the same side. The internal lining of the Fallopian tube contains many hairlike structures called *cilia*. The cilia are responsible for "sweeping" the egg down the tube after ovulation.

67. *What are the fimbria of the Fallopian tube?*

The fimbria are fingerlike projections at the end of each Fallopian tube that cover the ovary at the time of ovulation. They enable the tube to "pick up" the egg so it can enter the tube. The fimbria must be free of scar tissue and adhesions, or it may be very difficult for you to become pregnant.

68. *What are ovaries?*

The ovaries are the sexual glands where eggs are formed. There are usually two ovaries—one on each side of the uterus. The ovaries also produce estrogen and progesterone and smaller amounts of testosterone. See illustration on page 32.

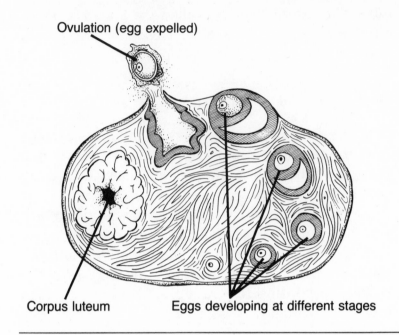

Ovulation (egg expelled)

Corpus luteum   Eggs developing at different stages

Ovary with developing eggs in the ovary, a corpus luteum and ovulation.

FSH and LH stimulate the ovaries. Estrogen and progesterone produced by the ovary stimulate the uterine lining to prepare it for implantation in the event pregnancy occurs.

69. *Do both ovaries function each month?*

Usually one ovary becomes the predominant ovary during a particular month. You may ovulate from your right ovary for several months in a row, then from the left ovary. Ovaries usually do not alternate on a regular basis.

70. *If I have only one ovary, does it mean I will ovulate every other month?*

No, you will still ovulate monthly. If only one ovary is present, it will produce an egg each month. You should still ovulate monthly with regular menstrual periods, if all the other glands and hormones function normally.

71. *What is the ovum?*

The ovum is the female reproductive cell also called the *egg*. It is expelled from the ovary at the time of ovulation. When fertilized by the sperm, the egg develops into an embryo, then a fetus.

72. *What is ovulation?*

Ovulation is the process by which the egg is expelled from the ovary and picked up by the Fallopian tube to begin its journey toward the uterus.

73. *What is the corpus luteum?*

It is a yellow mass formed by cells in the area of the ovary where the egg was emitted. A corpus luteum develops from the graafian follicle (the area that contains the egg) after ovulation occurs. It produces the hormone progesterone, which is needed to maintain a developing pregnancy.

If pregnancy occurs, the corpus luteum becomes a corpus luteum of pregnancy and is responsible for progesterone production during the first 3 months of pregnancy until the placenta takes over this function. If pregnancy does not occur, the corpus luteum gradually dissolves and disappears with the next menstrual cycle.

74. *What is a womb?*

A womb is a common term for the uterus.

75. *What is a tipped uterus?*

About 80% of all women have a uterus that is in the anterior position, which means the uterus faces the front of a woman's body. The other 20% have a uterus that is bent toward the back; it is called a *tipped uterus*.

76. *Does a tipped uterus cause infertility?*

This is an old wives' tale. If there are no other abnormalities of your organs, a tipped uterus does *not* mean a higher incidence of infertility.

77. *What is a hysterectomy?*

Hyster is Greek for uterus, and *ectomy* is Greek for removal. Hysterectomy means to surgically remove the uterus, including the cervix.

78. *What is a salpingectomy?*

Salpingo is Greek for tube. Salpingectomy means to surgically remove the Fallopian tube.

79. *What is an oophorectomy?*

Oophoros is Greek for ovary. Oophorectomy means to surgically remove the ovary. A *unilateral oophorectomy* means removal of one ovary; a *bilateral oophorectomy* means removal of both ovaries.

80. *When a woman has a hysterectomy, does it mean her ovaries and tubes are also removed?*

Usually it doesn't because hysterectomy means removal of only the uterus. If you have your uterus, both tubes and both ovaries removed, the procedure is called *hysterectomy plus a bilateral salpingoophorectomy*. If one ovary and tube are left, it is called a *unilateral salpingoophorectomy*.

MALE GENITAL SYSTEM

It's important for you to be familiar with the male reproduction system and male organs. The external parts of the male genitals include the penis and scrotum. Internal organs include the testicles, urethra, Cowper's glands, prostate gland, seminal vesicles and epididymis. See illustrations on pages 36 and 39.

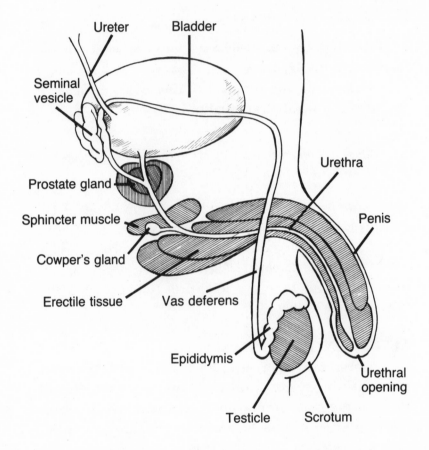

Male reproductive system.

81. *What is a testicle?*

It is an egg-shaped gland, located in the scrotum, that produces sperm and testosterone.

82. *What is the scrotum?*

It is a skin pouch that hangs between a man's legs and holds the testicles.

83. *Why are the testicles located outside the body?*

Testicles are very sensitive to body heat. Outside of the body cavity in the scrotal sac, testicles are at a temperature about 4 degrees lower than the normal body temperature. If testicles were located inside the abdominal cavity, they would be unable to produce sperm because of the increase in body temperature, which is incompatible with sperm production.

84. *How does the scrotum control the temperature of the testicles when outside temperature changes?*

The scrotum has the capability of expanding or contracting, depending on its exposure to heat or cold. When exposed to heat, the scrotum relaxes, and testicles fall and hang low in the scrotal sac. When exposed to cold, the scrotum contracts and draws the testicles closer to the body to warm them.

85. *Can a man voluntarily control this reflex?*

No; it's a reflex he can't control.

86. *Does anything else control the temperature of the testicles?*

The arteries and veins around the testicles help regulate their temperature. Too much blood around the testicles, which occurs in a varicocele, raises the temperature and interferes with sperm production.

87. *Why is temperature regulation important in sperm production?*

A very small rise in the temperature can affect the amount of sperm produced and how fast the sperm will move. A higher temperature inhibits sperm production and decreases the motility of sperm.

88. *In what part of the testicles are sperm produced?*

The testicles are made up of hundreds of tiny tubules called *seminiferous tubules.* Sperm are manufactured in these tubules, then come together into a smaller network called the *rete testis.* The tubules of the rete testis eventually come together into the epididymis, then into the vas deferens. The vas deferens ends in the urethra where sperm are ejaculated through the penis.

89. *How many testicles are there?*

Most men have two testicles—one on each side of the scrotum.

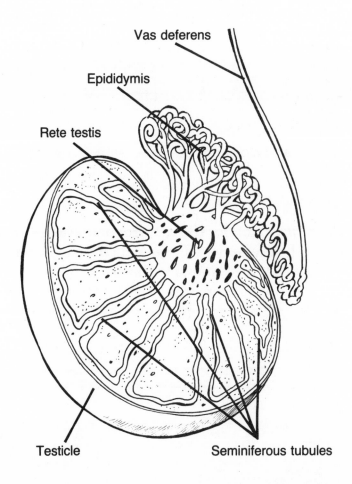

Vas deferens

Epididymis

Rete testis

Testicle

Seminiferous tubules

Cross section of testicle.

90. *Do some men only have one testicle?*

Yes. Occasionally a man is born with only one testicle or one must be removed for medical reasons, such as torsion or tumors.

91. *Does having only one testicle interfere with a man's fertility?*

If the testicle is normal, it will produce enough sperm and does not interfere with fertility.

92. *What is sperm?*

Sperm is short for spermatozoon, the male reproductive cell necessary to impregnate the egg. Each sperm has a head, neck and tail. The head and neck contain the genetic traits from the father. The tail is responsible for making the sperm move. See illustration below.

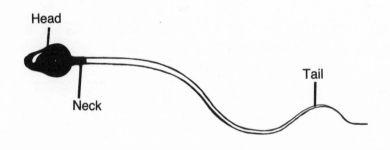

Sperm.

93. *What is testosterone?*

It is a hormone produced by the Leydig cells in the testicle. Testosterone is responsible for the development and growth of a man's sexual characteristics, which include the size of the penis, the development of pubic, axillary and facial hair, and deepening of the voice.

94. *What are Leydig cells?*

Leydig cells are located at the base of the seminiferous tubules within the testicle, and they produce testosterone.

95. *What hormones control production of sperm and testosterone by the testicles?*

FSH and LH control production of sperm and testosterone.

96. *What is the epididymis?*

The epididymis is a coiled, tubular structure located on top of the testicle. Sperm are stored there after they leave the seminiferous tubules and rete testis. If the epididymis was stretched out, it would be about 20 feet long. Sperm are stored at the tail end of the epididymis; at the time of ejaculation, sperm move into the vas deferens.

97. *Do sperm undergo any changes in the epididymis?*

Sperm that enter the epididymis from the testicle are unable to swim or move; they are incapable of fertilizing an egg. As they pass through the epididymis, sperm mature to become capable of fertilizing an egg. Sperm are stored at the end of the epididymis, awaiting ejaculation.

98. *What happens to sperm if they stay in the epididymis too long?*

They become old and lose their ability to fertilize.

99. *How can this interfere with conception?*

If a man decides to "save all his sperm" for intercourse once a month at midcycle, he actually decreases his chance of impregnating his wife. Most of the sperm are dead and inactive. It's best to have intercourse several times a month to prevent sperm from becoming "sluggish."

100. *How long does it take sperm to be produced?*

The whole process, from sperm production to ejaculation, takes about 72 days—sperm are manufactured in the seminiferous tubules, then migrate through the rete testis and mature in the epididymis.

101. *What happens to sperm if a man is exposed to a substance that interferes with sperm production?*

External factors, such as toxic chemicals or some medications, can affect sperm production at various stages of development. If exposure to a toxin occurs at the early stage of development, it may take 72 days for sperm production to return to normal after the substance is eliminated that caused the abnormality.

102. *How many sperm are released at one time?*

As many as 300 million sperm may be released in an ejaculate. Several hundred sperm may reach the Fallopian tube where the egg is located.

103. *What is an ejaculate?*

Ejaculate means to expel suddenly. In reference to a man, it also means the substance expelled when a man has an orgasm.

104. *What does the ejaculate contain?*

It contains sperm and seminal fluid. The first part of the ejaculate usually contains most of the sperm, and the second part of the ejaculate is chiefly fluid. Ejaculate can be separated when a man masturbates by having him catch the first part of the ejaculate in one container and the second part in another container. This takes a quick reaction!

105. *Are the contents of the ejaculate important?*

Yes. When a woman is artificially inseminated, it may be best to use the first part of the ejaculate because it usually contains most of the sperm. A "split" ejaculate semen analysis should be done to verify this.

106. *How many sperm fertilize an egg?*

It takes only one sperm to fertilize the egg. But even under totally normal circumstances, you only have a 15% chance during each cycle for pregnancy to occur.

Only a few sperm out of several million reach the Fallopian tube. Most of the sperm become immobilized in the vagina, cervix and uterus before entering the Fallopian tube. For reasons we do not fully understand, even if a sperm meets the egg in the Fallopian tube, it may not be capable of fertilizing the egg. When the sperm count is too low (below 20 million) or sperm motility is abnormal, no sperm may reach the Fallopian tube, making conception impossible.

107. *How long can sperm live?*

Sperm ejaculated into a specimen jar, such as when obtaining a specimen for analysis, can live from 2 to 8 hours. Sperm deposited into the vagina may live from 2 to 4 days. Sperm live longer in a "natural" environment, such as cervical or uterine mucus, because of nutritional, pH and environmental factors needed for survival compared to existing in a jar. There are reports that sperm have survived for as long as a week.

108. *What is semen?*

Semen is another term for the ejaculate—it contains seminal fluid and sperm.

109. *What is seminal fluid?*

It is the fluid secreted in an ejaculate that contains the nutrients that enable the sperm to survive after they are deposited in the vagina.

110. *Where does most of the fluid in an ejaculate come from?*

Most of the fluid comes from the prostate gland and two glands called the *seminal vesicles*.

111. *What are the seminal vesicles?*

They are a pair of glands located behind the urinary bladder in a man; these glands are responsible for most of the fluid in an ejaculation. During intercourse and ejaculation, the seminal glands forcefully expel their fluid behind the sperm, forcing the sperm out of the vas deferens, into the male urethra, where it is expelled into the vagina.

112. *What is the prostate gland?*

The prostate is a gland that surrounds the neck of the bladder and urethra. It secretes an important chemical that causes semen to liquefy after ejaculation. Liquefaction of semen is necessary so sperm can escape out of the seminal fluid into the cervical mucus.

113. *How can abnormalities of the prostate gland cause infertility?*

The prostate gland can be a common source of an infection called *prostatitis,* which is an inflammation of the prostate gland. Infection can be caused by gonorrhea, chlamydia or other bacteria.

The infection may cause a pus-filled secretion from the prostate gland and penis, which may alter the quality of the seminal fluid. Because the quality of the seminal fluid is poor, sperm may not survive or they may be incapable of fertilizing an egg.

114. *What are Cowper's glands?*

They are a pair of small glands located at the base of the penis that contribute a small amount of fluid to the ejaculate. The fluid provides additional nutrition needed by the sperm.

115. *What is the urethra?*

It is a membranous, tubelike structure that runs from the bladder, through the prostate gland and through the entire length of the penis. It has two main functions.

● It carries urine from the bladder to the outside of the body.

● During intercourse and ejaculation, it expels sperm and seminal fluid.

116. *What is a penis?*

It is the male sex organ that contains the urethra. It is made up of two parallel cylindrical tubes, called the *corpora cavernosa*. Beneath them is the corpus spongiosum, which contains the urethra. These structures contain many veins that fill with blood during sexual arousal. When blood fills these veins, an erection in the penis occurs, which allows the stiffened penis to enter the vagina.

117. *If the urethra carries semen and urine, does a man expel urine when he has an ejaculation?*

There is a special valve at the base of the bladder that closes at the time of ejaculation—this prevents urine from being released from the bladder. There is also a valve in the prostate gland that prevents seminal fluid from being released when a man urinates.

3

What Can We Do Before Seeking Medical Help?

Before you seek medical help as a couple for an infertility problem, there are a few things you can consider. Some are lifestyle changes; some are changes in your awareness level. The information in this section may help you understand what you can do for yourself to deal with this problem *before* seeking medical help.

1. *How does pregnancy occur?*

For pregnancy to occur, sperm must meet and fertilize an egg. This usually happens through sexual intercourse.

2. *What is intercourse?*

Intercourse means a mutual exchange. Sexual intercourse is the process in which the erect penis of the male is inserted into the vagina of the female. When ejaculation occurs in the male, sperm are deposited into the vagina.

3. *What happens after sperm are deposited in the vagina?*

Sperm enter the cervix and travel into the uterine cavity. They must find their way out of the uterus into the Fallopian tube, where they wait for an egg to be released from the ovary. If a sperm is able to penetrate the egg, pregnancy begins.

Penetration of the egg by the sperm is called *fertilization*. After 5 to 7 days, the fertilized egg gradually returns to the uterus where it embeds into the nutritious uterine lining and develops into an embryo.

4. *When is pregnancy most likely to occur?*

It doesn't matter for a man. For a woman, it depends on when she ovulates.

5. *What is ovulation?*

Ovulation is the process by which an egg is released from the ovary and swept into the Fallopian tube by the fimbria. Once in the Fallopian tube, the egg starts its journey toward the uterus, where it awaits fertilization by a sperm.

6. *What happens to the egg if pregnancy does not occur?*

The egg dissolves in the Fallopian tube or uterus and disappears.

7. *When does ovulation occur in most women?*

Most women are on a 28-to-32 day menstrual cycle. In predicting when you will probably ovulate, count the first day of your menstrual flow as day 1 of your cycle. A 28-day cycle means it is 28 days from the first day of menstrual flow to the first day of the next menstrual flow.

The time from ovulation until your *next* period is the most predictable time of your cycle. This is often 14 days. If you have a 28-day cycle, ovulation occurs about day 14 (28 - 14 = 14). If you have a 32-day cycle, ovulation will be on day 18 (32 - 14 = 18). If you have a 35-day cycle, ovulation will be on day 21.

8. *When is the best time of the month to have intercourse to achieve pregnancy?*

It's best to have sperm present in the Fallopian tube when ovulation occurs, so intercourse should not only occur at the time of ovulation but also *before* ovulation. This is best accomplished by having intercourse every other day around the time of ovulation.

Ovulation time is often called *midcycle time*. Begin having intercourse around day 10 of your cycle and continue every other day for the next 6 to 10 days, depending on the length of your cycle.

9. *Can we have intercourse during other parts of the cycle?*

Having intercourse throughout the menstrual cycle is normal and acceptable. It won't decrease your chance for pregnancy.

10. *Why should we have intercourse every other day?*

Intercourse on a daily basis may be fine for many

couples. But a man with a borderline sperm count may benefit from the extra day of rest to allow the sperm count to recover to a normal range.

11. *What about saving sperm for ovulation day and having intercourse only once or twice a month?*

Infrequent intercourse, such as only a few times a month, *decreases* the sperm's motility and may decrease your chance to conceive. This can be important in some cases of infertility. In general, it's best to have intercourse a few times a week, not only at the time of ovulation.

12. *How long do sperm live?*

Most sperm live 48 to 72 hours. Occasionally, sperm may live up to 1 week and still be capable of fertilizing an egg.

13. *How long does the egg live?*

The egg is much less durable than the sperm and lives for only 12 to 24 hours. Because of the short time in which the egg can be fertilized, it's best to have sperm waiting for the egg in the Fallopian tube at the time of ovulation.

14. *How long does it normally take a couple to become pregnant?*

Assuming everything is normal with both partners, the average time to achieve pregnancy is 4 to 6 months. About 1 in 4 couples achieve pregnancy within the first month of trying, and 85% achieve pregnancy within the first year.

15. *What if I have an extremely long cycle?*

If your cycle is about 38 days, it means you are ovulating on day 24 of your cycle. In this case, have intercourse at least through day 25 of your cycle or until your temperature is elevated on your BBT (basal body temperature). If your cycle is irregular or longer than this, you may be a candidate for an ovulation-inducing drug, such as clomiphene citrate.

16. *What if I have an extremely short cycle?*

Some women have a very short cycle, such as 23 days. This means ovulation occurs about day 9 of the cycle. In this case, intercourse should start as early as day 7 to ensure the presence of sperm when ovulation occurs.

17. *When is an extremely short cycle important in becoming pregnant?*

In certain religions, such as Orthodox Judaism, intercourse is not allowed until 7 days after menstruation has stopped. If a woman flows for 5 to 6 days and ovulates on day 9 or 10, it means intercourse will not occur until *after* ovulation. It would be impossible to become pregnant if this is practiced on a regular basis.

18. *How can I be sure if ovulation is occurring?*

You can record your basal body temperature (BBT).

19. *What does basal mean?*

It means the body is at total rest.

20. *What is a basal body temperature recording?*

It is a daily recording of your temperature the first thing in the morning, before you get out of bed.

21. *How is this done?*

Your temperature is taken and recorded daily and placed on a graph. After a month has passed, you can look at the graph to see what has happened.

Normally, the body temperature is about 98.6F (37C). In actuality, the morning temperature before ovulation is below 98F (36.5C). It may be as low as 97F (36.1C).

After ovulation, the basal temperature is often just above 98F (36.6C). This shift in temperature indicates ovulation on a temperature graph. See illustrations on pages 54 and 55.

22. *Why does the temperature change?*

After ovulation, the area in the ovary that expelled the egg becomes a corpus luteum. The corpus luteum secretes progesterone, which causes the temperature-control area in the hypothalmus to raise the body's temperature.

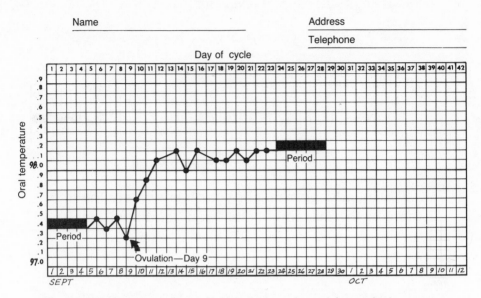

Basal-temperature chart for 23-day cycle, with ovulation on Day 9.

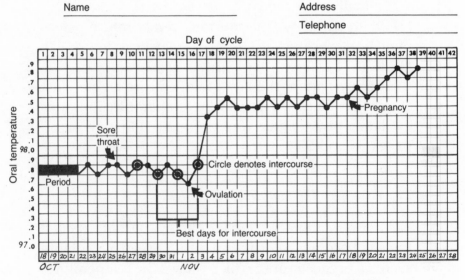

Basal-temperature chart for 28-day cycle, with pregnancy. (Circle denotes intercourse.) Once temperature remains elevated for longer than 16 days, pregnancy is strongly suggested.

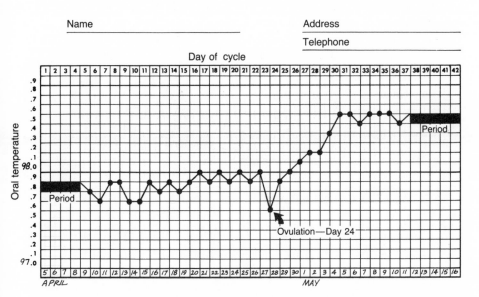

Basal-temperature chart for 38-day cycle, with ovulation on Day 24.

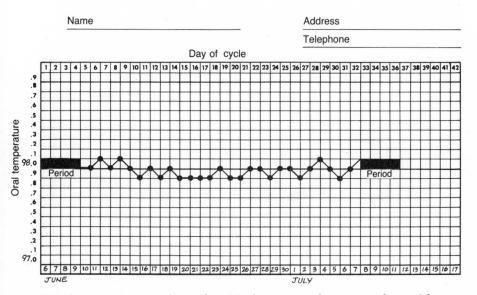

Basal-temperature chart for 32-day anovulatory cycle, with no ovulation.

23. *When should I start to record my basal body temperature?*

It is usually not necessary for everyone to start recording a BBT when trying to achieve pregnancy. If you have a regular cycle of 26 to 34 days, which is preceded by premenstrual symptoms of breast tenderness, occasional moodiness and water-weight gain, it usually means you are ovulating.

24. *When is a BBT helpful?*

Recording your BBT is most helpful if your cycles are irregular or if you don't become pregnant after trying for 6 months. Recording a BBT is useful if you take any type of ovulation-inducing medication.

25. *What are the functions of a basal-temperature graph?*

It can give the approximate day you ovulated, and it helps in scheduling tests that are performed during an infertility investigation. BBT also helps determine the length of the pre- and post-ovulatory part of your menstrual cycle.

26. *Can a man record his basal body temperature?*

He can, but it is basically the same all month long and has no purpose in trying to achieve pregnancy.

27. *Is there a special thermometer to use to take my BBT?*

A basal thermometer is available. It records temperatures between 96 and 100F (35.5 and 37.5C). The markings are farther apart so it is easier to read than a regular thermometer.

28. *Where can I purchase a basal thermometer?*

Most drugstores sell basal thermometers; they cost about $8.

29. *It is necessary to use a basal thermometer to record a BBT?*

No, it isn't. A regular thermometer can be used. It may be slightly more difficult to read, but it is usually satisfactory.

30. *How do I take my basal temperature?*

1. Shake down the thermometer before you go to bed at night.
2. Immediately after you wake up, before you get out of bed, put the thermometer under your tongue for 5 minutes.
3. Read the thermometer to the nearest 0.10 of a degree.
4. Chart your temperature on the graph that comes with the thermometer, or make your own chart.
5. If you have a cold, sore throat or aren't feeling well, take your temperature, record it and note on the graph your problem.
6. Circle the days you have intercourse on the graph.

31. *Why is it important to take my temperature before getting out of bed?*

Even a slight amount of activity, such as getting up to go to the bathroom, will cause a slight rise in the basal temperature. You are looking for only a 0.6 degree change, so it's important to take your temperature *before* any activity.

32. *Will my temperature change if I get up earlier or later than usual?*

There may be a slight change, but one day isn't critical. It's the general pattern of a lower temperature during the first part of the cycle and a higher temperature during the latter part of the cycle that is important.

33. *What happens if I forget to take my temperature for 1 or 2 days?*

One or two temperatures are not as important as the pattern for the whole month, so there's no need for concern.

34. *What does a normal graph look like?*

The basal temperature is usually below 98F (36.5C) during the first half of the cycle. Just before ovulation, there may be a slight dip, then a rise in the temperature. It stays up until menstruation occurs then falls back to the range of the first part of the cycle. The difference between the first part and the second part of the cycle is usually 0.6 to 0.8 of a degree.

35. *Can I tell the exact time of ovulation, according to my temperatures?*

Ovulation occurs *just before* the temperature starts to rise. Often there is a slight dip in the temperature before the rise. If there is a dip, ovulation is probably at that point.

You may not be able to tell the exact day you ovulate but should be able to tell within a 2-to-3-day period. The exact point of ovulation can't always be determined from looking at a graph, especially if the temperature rise is erratic.

36. *When should we have intercourse to become pregnant?*

A temperature graph can't tell you when to have intercourse during the current cycle. Many women are under the impression they must wait for the temperature rise, then have intercourse. *If you do this, it is too late to become pregnant during that cycle!*

The BBT can be used as a guide to the time to have intercourse during the *next* cycle by giving the *approximate* day of ovulation. Intercourse should occur every other day around ovulation time for the best chance of pregnancy. Intercourse should occur before the temperature rise not after the rise. *Once the temperature is on the rise, it's too late to become pregnant during that cycle!*

37. *What if my temperature stays elevated, and I don't get my period?*

It usually means you're pregnant. In fact, if you're taking your BBT, a persistently elevated temperature is one of the first indications you are pregnant. If the temperature stays elevated for at least 16 days after the rise, it is very likely you are pregnant.

38. *What else can a temperature chart show?*

It can indicate if you have a condition called a *luteal phase defect* in which there is a very short interval between ovulation and your next period.

39. *What causes this short interval?*

The luteal phase defect is usually caused by a deficiency of progesterone, which is produced by the corpus luteum of the ovary. There are several ways to treat luteal phase defects, including the use of clomiphene citrate, human chorionic gonadotropin or progesterone. See page 94.

40. *Are there other symptoms that tell me if I'm ovulating?*

Most women can't tell when they ovulate. Occasionally, you may get low abdominal pain, which lasts from a few minutes to a few hours, at the time of ovulation; this is called *mittleschmerz.*

41. *What causes mittleschmerz?*

It is the result of a small amount of fluid or blood that escapes from the ovary at the time of ovulation.

42. *Are there other signs of ovulation?*

Some woman have a large amount of watery discharge from the vagina. The discharge comes from the cervical glands and peaks at ovulation time; it may be associated with minimal spotting.

43. *Are there other tests that help determine the time of ovulation?*

Several tests are available for home use; they have the capability of predicting ovulation *before* it occurs.

44. *What kind of tests are they?*

They are urine tests that use monoclonal-antibody technology to measure LH in your urine. Before ovulation, there is a sudden rise in LH in the bloodstream, and it is excreted into your urine. It is believed that by determining when this occurs is the best way of determining *impending* ovulation.

45. *How soon after the rise in LH does ovulation occur?*

There is an extremely sharp rise of LH about 12 to 36 hours before ovulation. LH can be measured in the urine with one of these tests.

46. *What are the names of these tests?*

The names of tests now available are OvuStick Self-Test, First Response Ovulation Predictor Test and OvuTime. They are all basically the same. Other tests similar to these will probably become available as different companies begin to manufacture them.

47. *How do I use one of these tests?*

You must do a series of urine tests each morning for several consecutive days. It's similar to a home pregnancy test, and it's fairly simple to use. Directions come with the kit.

Strips of paper included in the kit show a marked change in color as LH rises. Once the color change occurs, ovulation will occur within the *next* 12 to 36 hours. Because there is a delay from the peak of LH to ovulation, it allows you to time intercourse or artificial insemination.

48. *Should we use this test?*

This test is helpful if you have an irregular cycle and are having difficulty with timed intercourse. It's also helpful in timing artificial insemination and scheduling endometrial biopsies. The test can help reduce the number of artificial inseminations for each cycle.

49. *How expensive are these tests?*

At this time, they are fairly expensive. They cost $25 to $65 a kit; each kit is good for 6 to 9 tests depending on the test used. As they become more popular, prices will probably drop.

These tests may be used for routine screening of ovulation, but it may not be necessary if you are having regular cycles and no fertility problem. Their only disadvantage is their cost. For routine screening, the BBT is still satisfactory for documenting ovulation in most women.

50. *What if I have difficulty with the test?*

Instructions are very complete. If you have problems, a toll-free number is included so you can call for answers to your questions.

51. *Where can I buy these tests?*

OvuStick is available by prescription from your doctor. First Response and OvuTime are sold over-the-counter in drugstores. Some doctors have tests available in their offices.

52. *Is one position during intercourse better than another when trying to become pregnant?*

The "missionary position," with the man on top and the woman below, is considered the best position. If the woman is on top, semen may leak out of the vagina before it can enter the cervix.

53. *Should artificial lubricants be used when trying to become pregnant?*

No, they should not. Vaseline and K-Y jelly can kill sperm and should not be used.

54. *What can be done about lubrication during intercourse?*

Most of the time, poor lubrication during intercourse results from not enough sexual foreplay. Allow plenty of time for arousal—don't rush to achieve male orgasm.

55. *What is an orgasm?*

It is the last stage of sexual excitement.

56. *What happens when orgasm occurs in a man?*

Orgasm results in the ejaculation of seminal fluid and sperm from the penis.

57. *What happens when orgasm occurs in a woman?*

Orgasm results in rhythmic contractions of the vagina, uterus and pelvic muscles, followed by total relaxation.

58. *Does orgasm have to occur for pregnancy to occur?*

Sperm can leak out of the penis before ejaculation occurs, so it's not impossible, but it's unlikely you'll become pregnant without a male orgasm. This is the reason withdrawal of the penis from the vagina does not always work for birth control.

In a woman, an orgasm is definitely *not* needed to become pregnant.

59. *Are there intercourse techniques that may be helpful or harmful?*

Yes, there are. Don't get up to urinate or douche immediately following intercourse. It may be best to lie in bed on your back or side for 15 to 20 minutes following intercourse. This prevents sperm from leaking out of the vagina. Some doctors suggest placing a pillow under your hips during intercourse to make it easier for sperm to get into the cervical canal.

60. *Will having timed intercourse have an effect on our enjoyment of sex?*

Unfortunately, following a rigid timing for intercourse may take the enjoyment out of sex. It may cause impotence in the man and lack of desire for sex in a couple. If this occurs, it may be best to take a "break" from trying to conceive for a few months.

61. *Are there other causes of infertility that I should be concerned about?*

There are many different things that may cause mild changes in your body that may influence your ability to conceive. Your general health, diet, stress, exercise pattern, personal habits and any medications you take may have some influence on fertility. Lubricants used during intercourse may also interfere.

62. *Can my state of health affect my fertility?*

You should be in good general health before you try to conceive. Many different organs of the body must function normally for conception to occur, so it is wise not to have severe medical problems when trying to get pregnant.

63. *Can poor nutrition cause infertility?*

If your weight is stable and you eat normally, diet should not be a factor. Severe malnutrition and rapid weight loss may cause you to stop ovulating, which causes you to become infertile. A man's sperm count may become abnormal if he is malnourished.

64. *Does stress cause infertility?*

Extremely severe stress can cause your menstrual cycle to become irregular and ovulation to cease. Severe stress in a man may cause difficulty during intercourse; impotence may result. Lesser degrees of stress and worrying about becoming pregnant may have some influence on fertility, but this is not fully understood at this time.

65. *Is it true many women become pregnant after adopting a child?*

Some infertile women become pregnant after adopting a child but probably no more than infertile women in the general population. Many people feel once a child is adopted, the pressure is off, which makes it easier for a couple to conceive.

66. *Can exercise interfere with becoming pregnant?*

Exercise on a regular basis is *excellent* for your health and general well-being. A normal exercise program, if not overly done, does not interfere with becoming pregnant.

67. *What if the exercise is done to extreme?*

It is not uncommon for women who exercise to extreme, such as marathon training, to develop irregular periods or amenorrhea. A woman's body fat plays an important role in estrogen production, with subsequent effect on the production of FSH and LH. If you are extremely underweight for any reason, you may not be ovulating—your periods may be irregular or absent, which would result in infertility.

In men, excessive exercise has little effect unless a man has a borderline semen analysis. In that case, extreme exercise may suppress the sperm count or decrease the sperm's motility.

68. *What should I do if extreme exercise causes infertility?*

Curtail exercise, and gain up to your ideal body weight. Limit running to under 20 miles a week. Once you cut down on your running and gain weight, your periods and ovulation should return to normal. In men with borderline sperm production, a gradual improvement in sperm count should occur.

69. *Does alcohol have an effect on infertility?*

Alcohol can affect fertility in several ways. In a man, it may interfere with maintaining an erection. With chronic alcohol use, a man may have decreased testosterone levels and decreased sperm production. Occasional social drinking should not have much of an effect.

In women, chronic use of alcohol may reduce the output of pituitary hormones and cause a woman to have irregular menstrual cycles. In men and women, chronic use of alcohol can affect hormone production because of interference with the liver. When you are trying to become pregnant, it's best to avoid excessive amounts of alcohol. An occasional drink should do no harm, but once pregnant, avoid alcohol.

70. *Does cigarette smoking affect fertility?*

Cigarette smoking and nicotine probably do not affect your ability to conceive. But smoking may increase the risk of miscarriage and interfere with fetal growth and development once pregnancy occurs. Heavy smoking doubles the miscarriage rate. The risks are even greater if there are already other high risk factors present, such as diabetes or high blood pressure.

Heavy smoking decreases the blood supply to the placenta and may result in a smaller birth-weight baby. There is a 30 to 50% risk of growth retardation of a fetus in a mother who smokes heavily. Smoking may also increase chances for certain pregnancy complications in the mother, such as premature separation of the placenta.

Women who stop smoking by the beginning of their fourth month of pregnancy may not have any increased risk over non-smokers. It's never too late to stop smoking during pregnancy!

71. *Does smoking affect fertility in a man?*

In a man with a borderline semen analysis, smoking may further depress the sperm quality. It's best if neither of you smoke when trying to conceive.

72. *Do pipe and cigar smoking affect fertility?*

Pipe and cigar smoking have the same impact as cigarette smoking because the effects of smoking are related to nicotine. Nicotine is a vasoconstrictor that decreases the blood supply to the uterus.

73. *Does marijuana affect fertility?*

It depends on the amount that is consumed. Small amounts, used very occasionally, probably do not have much of an effect except in someone with an additional reproductive problem.

In women, large amounts of marijuana can decrease the production of FSH, LH and prolactin. This may cause irregular periods and cessation of ovulation.

In men, large amounts of marijuana may decrease testosterone levels and inhibit sperm production and motility.

74. *Does cocaine affect fertility?*

Cocaine use is believed to increase the chance of a spontaneous miscarriage. Preliminary studies also suggest an increased incidence of cryptorchidism (undescended testicles) and kidney abnormalities to the fetus if it is exposed to cocaine in the first few weeks following conception, even with minimal exposure.

Babies born to mothers who used cocaine may also have a higher incidence of Sudden Infant Death Syndrome (SIDS) and later learning disabilities.

If you are trying to conceive, *don't* use cocaine!

75. *What is DES?*

DES (diethylstilbestrol) is a synthetic estrogen first developed in the 1930s. During the 1940s and '50s, many physicians prescribed it to pregnant women with complications of pregnancy, such as bleeding, threatened miscarriage or diabetes. DES was used to try to prevent miscarriages and improve the outcome of the pregnancy.

76. *What problems have been associated with exposure to DES?*

Some children born to mothers who took DES during pregnancy have been found to have abnormalities with their genital and reproductive organs. Some daughters have had abnormalities of the vagina, cervix, uterus and Fallopian tubes. There is an increase in infertility, and once pregnant, miscarriage rates are higher in these women. Recently, sons who were exposed have also been shown to have abnormalities of their ductal system with an increased incidence of semen abnormalities that can cause infertility.

77. *What should I do if I was exposed to DES?*

Consult your doctor to see if any abnormalities are present. Often a routine pelvic exam or semen analysis can determine if there is an effect from DES exposure.

78. *Do other medications and chemicals affect fertility?*

Many different medications may affect fertility, especially sperm production. If you take *any* medicine, check with your doctor about possible effects. Some common over-the-counter antihistamines are known to cause a decrease in sperm production and motility.

4

What Do We Need to Know About Pregnancy?

If you are experiencing infertility, you are concerned about many aspects of the problem. Looking at the whole picture and understanding more about the condition of pregnancy may help you understand more about the problems you are having.

1. *What is pregnancy?*

Pregnancy is the condition of a developing embryo or fetus growing in a woman's body. It is the result of the union of the egg from a woman and sperm from a man, which is called *fertilization*.

2. *Where does fertilization take place?*

It takes place in the Fallopian tube.

3. *What happens after fertilization?*

During the first week after fertilization, the fertilized egg, now called a *morula*, begins to divide and multiply as it works its way down the Fallopian tube toward the uterus to enter the uterine cavity. The morula then implants itself into the uterine lining (endometrium) and begins further development.

4. *What happens to the ovary after ovulation occurs?*

The area in the ovary that contained the egg changes into the corpus luteum, which produces progesterone. Progesterone plays an important part in your menstrual cycle and prepares the uterine lining for implantation. Without progesterone, a fertilized egg would be unable to implant in the uterine lining. If you become pregnant, the corpus luteum becomes a corpus luteum of pregnancy.

5. *What is the function of a corpus luteum of pregnancy?*

The corpus luteum produces progesterone for the first 12 weeks of pregnancy. Once pregnancy occurs, progesterone is needed to nourish the uterine lining and support the pregnancy. If progesterone is removed (by removing the corpus luteum) during the first 3 months of pregnancy, a miscarriage will occur. After 3 months, the placenta takes over production of progesterone for the remainder of the pregnancy.

6. *How do I know if I'm pregnant?*

The most common symptoms of early pregnancy are a missed period, morning nausea, breast tenderness and a feeling of tiredness. If you are taking your basal body temperature at the time you conceive and your temperature remains elevated for more than 16 days, it is likely you are pregnant.

7. *What tests can determine if I am pregnant?*

The most common test is a urine pregnancy test. A pregnancy test measures the amount of HCG in the urine. HCG is secreted by the early developing placenta cells soon after implantation. Blood pregnancy tests can also be done.

8. *How soon can these tests determine if I am pregnant?*

Most tests doctors do in their offices and home pregnancy tests can determine pregnancy within 5 to 10 days after a missed period. Recently, more-sensitive urine tests have been developed that can determine if you are pregnant at the time of, or even before, a missed period.

Early tests may be done for a woman who is very anxious to find out if she is pregnant. Tests may also be used in cases in which it is important to determine if the woman is pregnant, such as following an abortion or a molar pregnancy, when certain drugs may be prescribed or if X-rays are needed. Occasionally it is necessary to determine if a woman is having "early miscarriages" rather than failing to become pregnant.

9. *How long will I have to wait for the results of a pregnancy test?*

Most pregnancy tests take only a few minutes. The more-sensitive blood or urine tests may take a few hours.

10. *Are home pregnancy tests accurate?*

Most home pregnancy tests are accurate. They may not be able to determine pregnancy as early as tests at your doctor's office, but they should be positive when you are 5 to 10 days late with your period. As newer tests are developed, they will be able to determine pregnancy earlier than tests now available.

11. *Can a pregnancy test be wrong?*

Yes, it can. All pregnancy tests have a small incidence (usually less than 2%) of false-positives (positive when a woman is not pregnant) or false-negatives (negative when a woman is pregnant).

12. *Where can I buy a home pregnancy tests?*

Most drugstores sell them.

13. *Can my doctor perform any other tests to determine if I am pregnant?*

By doing a pelvic examination, your doctor may be able to see if your cervix has turned slightly blue and if the uterus is softer and slightly enlarged. Approximately 10 weeks beyond a missed period, it may be possible to hear the fetal heart beat with an ultrasound stethoscope. An ultrasound exam may be necessary if there is concern about a possible miscarriage or ectopic pregnancy.

14. *How do multiple pregnancies occur?*

Twins can occur in two different ways. In one instance, two different eggs are fertilized by two different sperm. These twins are called *fraternal* or *non-identical twins*. They come from two different eggs and sperm, so the babies born have different genes.

In the second instance, a fertilized egg splits in two early in its development. The splitting occurs after the egg is fertilized and before it implants into the uterus. These are identical twins because they come from the same fertilized egg. They have the same genetic makeup.

15. *How frequent are multiple pregnancies?*

Twins occur in about 1 in 86 pregnancies under normal conditions. Triplets occur in about 1 in 7,000 to 8,000 pregnancies.

16. *Do fertility drugs increase my chance of having a multiple pregnancy?*

Yes! When Clomid is used to achieve pregnancy, twins occur in 6 to 8% of all pregnancies. With Pergonal, twins occur 20 to 30% of the time. Pergonal is the drug usually taken when you read about a woman having four, five, six or even seven babies.

If you need an ovulation-inducing drug, such as Clomid or Pergonal, the effect of the drug lasts only during that cycle. If you take Clomid and have twins, you are not at higher risk for twins with the second pregnancy, unless you take Clomid again. But if you have only one baby with the first pregnancy, you could have twins with the second pregnancy.

17. *What is an ectopic pregnancy?*

An ectopic pregnancy is one that implants and grows someplace other than in the uterus.

18. *Where is the most common location for an ectopic pregnancy?*

The most common place outside the uterus is the Fallopian tube. This is called a *tubal pregnancy.*

19. *Where else can an ectopic pregnancy implant?*

A pregnancy can implant on the ovary, in the ligaments around the uterus, in the cervix or in the abdominal cavity. See illustration on page 78.

20. *What causes an ectopic pregnancy?*

Often we can't give a good explanation as to why an ectopic pregnancy occurs. However, there is an increase in the occurrence if Fallopian tubes have been damaged from infections, endometriosis or tubal surgery.

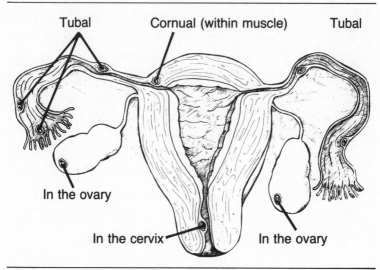

Various sites of ectopic pregnancies.

21. *What happens in an ectopic pregnancy?*

The fertilized egg implants in a place other than the uterus. As the egg starts to develop, it becomes larger and causes pressure on the structure it is developing around. This usually results in pain and possibly abnormal vaginal bleeding.

22. *What are the symptoms of ectopic pregnancy?*

The most common symptoms are a missed period, vaginal spotting and abdominal pain. If intra-abdominal bleeding occurs from a leakage of blood from a ruptured ectopic pregnancy, additional symptoms may be present. These include:

● Lightheadedness (feeling faint).

• Shoulder pain (from blood under the diaphragm and referred to the shoulder by the phrenic nerve).

• An urge to have a bowel movement.

The urge to have a bowel movement results from blood in the pelvis causing pressure on the rectum. It is not unusual for a woman to go into the bathroom and pass out from internal bleeding from a ruptured ectopic pregnancy. By being aware of early symptoms, hopefully most early ectopic pregnancies can be diagnosed *before* they rupture.

23. *Is an ectopic pregnancy dangerous?*

It can be a very dangerous complication of pregnancy. If you suspect you are pregnant and you develop these symptoms, contact your doctor immediately, or go to the emergency room of a hospital for evaluation and treatment!

24. *How is an ectopic pregnancy diagnosed?*

The symptoms of a missed period, a positive pregnancy test, vaginal spotting and abdominal pain should make a doctor suspicious of an ectopic pregnancy.

25. *Does every woman who has an ectopic pregnancy develop these symptoms?*

Occasionally a woman doesn't develop these early symptoms but will have severe abdominal pain, weakness, fainting and even shock from internal bleeding.

26. *Do symptoms of ectopic pregnancy resemble those of a possible miscarriage?*

Yes. That's why it's important to be examined so your doctor can determine if it is an ectopic pregnancy or a possible miscarriage.

27. *Can the doctor tell the difference?*

Even after an examination, it's sometimes difficult to tell the difference. Your doctor may want to use ultrasound to see if he can find where the pregnancy is developing. Laparoscopy may be necessary to determine if a pregnancy is developing outside the uterus. It's best to diagnose an ectopic pregnancy before it ruptures to prevent internal bleeding. See page 121.

28. *How is an ectopic pregnancy treated?*

It depends on where it is located. Ectopic pregnancy usually requires surgery with an abdominal incision. If the pregnancy is located in the Fallopian tube, it may be possible to make an incision in the tube, remove the developing pregnancy and repair the tube. If this is not possible, the tube may have to be removed.

A pregnancy implanted on an ovary may require removal of the ovary. A D&C may be done to remove a pregnancy located in the cervical canal. If bleeding from a cervical pregnancy cannot be controlled with a D&C, hysterectomy may be necessary.

Occasionally a tubal pregnancy is spontaneously expelled from the end of the Fallopian tube and can be removed by laparoscopy.

29. *How common is ectopic pregnancy?*

Ectopic pregnancies occur in about 1% of all pregnancies.

30. *Is it possible to have a twin pregnancy in which one is ectopic?*

It is possible to have a combined twin ectopic pregnancy or even a combined intrauterine and ectopic pregnancy, but these are extremely rare.

31. *Can an ectopic pregnancy be carried to full term?*

It is possible for the pregnancy to go to full term if the implantation occurs within the abdominal cavity or on the intestines, where the pregnancy has room to expand. This is a *very rare,* dangerous situation. Most doctors have never seen an abdominal pregnancy.

32. *What is a miscarriage?*

A miscarriage is the unanticipated, spontaneous loss of the fetus or placenta before the 20th week of pregnancy.

33. *What causes a miscarriage?*

If a pregnancy is not progressing normally, the lining of the uterus may break away from its attachment, shed and end the pregnancy. The medical terminology for a miscarriage is a *spontaneous abortion*. A naturally occurring miscarriage should not be confused with a planned therapeutic abortion, which is a voluntary procedure.

34. *How many pregnancies end in miscarriage?*

At least 15 to 20% of all pregnancies that continue beyond a missed menstrual period end in miscarriage.

35. *When do most miscarriages occur?*

A miscarriage can occur at any time during the first half of pregnancy, but 85% of them occur within the first 3 months. If a pregnancy loss occurs after the 20th week of pregnancy, it is called a *premature delivery* rather than a miscarriage.

36. *Is it important to see your doctor after a miscarriage?*

Yes, it is. Even if you feel you have miscarried completely, it is important to see your doctor because he needs to determine if there is any evidence of infection or retained tissue as a result of the miscarriage. If you have Rh-negative blood, you may need RhoD immune globulin (RhoGam) to prevent problems with Rh sensitization in future pregnancies.

37. *Do current pregnancy tests affect the miscarriage rate?*

The more-sensitive pregnancy tests can now detect pregnancy at the time of, or even before, a missed menstrual period. If these tests are used to detect pregnancy before a missed period, it's believed the miscarriage rate could be as high as 30 to 40% of all conceptions. In other words, when a woman has a very heavy period or is a "few days late" with her period, she may have been pregnant and had a very early miscarriage without knowing it.

38. *What causes most miscarriages?*

Most miscarriages occur because a developing pregnancy is not progressing normally. Some view it as Nature's way of taking care of an imperfect implantation. Most miscarriages are caused by a genetic mix-up in the growing embryo during its early stages of development.

39. *What causes this mix-up?*

Research indicates there is no apparent reason why the genetic mix-up occurs. These are random accidents that usually do not repeat themselves.

40. *Is there a formed fetus in most miscarriages?*

The genetic mix-up is not compatible with fetal development, so a formed fetus is *not* usually present in most miscarriages. The medical terminology for most early miscarriages is a *blighted ovum* or *empty-sac syndrome.*

41. *Can illness during pregnancy cause a miscarriage?*

Any severe illness associated with a temperature of 103 to 104F (39 to 40C) can be detrimental to fetal development and may lead to miscarriage or premature delivery. Illnesses, such as pneumonia, typhoid fever and pyelonephritis, have been associated with spontaneous miscarriages. Low-grade fevers from a common cold usually do no harm.

42. *What are other causes of miscarriage?*

Infections, abnormalities of the uterus and certain teratogens, such as radiation, drugs and chemicals, can cause a woman to miscarry. (A teratogen is any substance that can cause abnormal formation or development.)

43. *Is there always an explanation for a miscarriage?*

Despite what is known about miscarriages, often there is no explanation for the cause of a miscarriage.

44. *If fetal development never occurred, what is expelled at the time of a miscarriage?*

The developing membranes, placenta and uterine lining are expelled.

45. *Do miscarriages often occur again?*

Miscarriages caused by blighted ovum usually do not happen again. These miscarriages have no greater chance of recurring than if you have never had a miscarriage. Occasionally a woman will have repeated miscarriages.

46. *Can emotional stress cause me to miscarry?*

Researchers do not believe stress causes a woman to miscarry.

47. *Can lifting or other physical activity cause a miscarriage?*

Physical activity and exercise do *not* cause a miscarriage. Even if bleeding occurs after exercise and you miscarry, it is believed by most doctors the miscarriage was not related to the exercise.

48. *Does sexual intercourse cause a miscarriage?*

No. Intercourse does *not* cause miscarriage.

49. *What are the symptoms of a miscarriage?*

There are two symptoms—vaginal bleeding and cramping pain. The bleeding may be very light or similar to a menstrual period. The cramping often comes and goes and is usually stronger than menstrual cramps.

50. *Is all bleeding in early pregnancy a sign of an impending miscarriage?*

No. At the beginning of pregnancy, some women have slight bleeding when the fertilized egg implants into the uterine lining. This is called *implantation bleeding*, and a woman might think it was her period.

51. *What percentage of women experience bleeding?*

About 25 to 30% of all women have some degree of bleeding during the first 3 months of pregnancy. About half the time, the bleeding stops, and the pregnancy goes on without increased risk to mother or fetus. The other half of the women who bleed eventually miscarry.

52. *Will I miscarry if I have heavy bleeding and severe cramps?*

If you have heavy bleeding and severe cramps, you will probably miscarry.

53. *Can anything be done to prevent a miscarriage?*

In the past, doctors treated women with hospitalization, bed rest and hormonal medication in an attempt to prevent miscarriage. Studies have shown pregnancies that would have continued would have done so without medication and bed rest.

Pregnancies that would have failed did fail, despite treatment. Unless a specific reason can be found for your miscarriage, there is usually no treatment.

54. *Did medications given to prevent miscarriages cause harm?*

Yes. The most commonly prescribed medication was diethylstilbestrol, commonly called *DES*. Many girls born to mothers who received this medication have developed abnormalities of their vagina, cervix and uterus, with a decreased fertility rate. These young women are also at a slightly increased risk of developing malignancies of their cervix and vagina.

More recently, boys born to mothers who took DES during pregnancy have been found to have abnormalities of their vas deferens and epididymis, with a decreased fertility rate. Mothers who took the medication were not harmed—only their developing babies.

55. *Can I have a menstrual period and still be pregnant?*

Yes, you can. A lighter-than-normal period is relatively common during the first month of pregnancy. Occasionally, you may have several menstrual periods with a normally developing pregnancy.

56. *Where is the bleeding from?*

Bleeding usually comes from the area in the uterus where the pregnancy is not implanted. We do not know why a woman would continue to have menstrual bleeding with her pregnancy. Bleeding is probably related to the hormonal changes and the way the uterine lining reacts to these changes.

57. *Once bleeding occurs, are there any tests to determine if a miscarriage will occur?*

Yes, there are. Ultrasound during the first 3 months of pregnancy may help determine the outcome of the pregnancy. About 8 to 9 weeks from the last menstrual period, an ultrasound exam should show a developing fetus with a heartbeat.

This means fetal development has occurred, and chances for a miscarriage are less than 5%, even if bleeding is present. If the ultrasound examination shows an "empty sac" or a sac filled with blood, it's a sign the pregnancy will not continue; the chances for a miscarriage are almost 100%.

58. *What if a fetus is not developing?*

You and your doctor will have to make a decision about what to do. If you are bleeding very heavily or cramping severely, it would be best to perform a D&C or suction curettage. If you are not having severe cramping or bleeding, it may be best to repeat the ultrasound in a week to see if there is any change in the size of the sac or if fetal activity has developed. It is possible conception occurred 1 to 2 weeks later than originally believed and fetal development has not yet occurred.

59. *What is a D&C?*

D&C means *dilatation and curettage*. Dilatation is the process of opening the cervix with dilators to allow a spoon-shaped instrument, a *curette*, into the uterus to scrape out tissue. It is used to treat incomplete miscarriages and to diagnose and treat other causes of abnormal uterine bleeding.

60. *What is a suction curettage?*

Suction curettage is another way to empty the uterus following a miscarriage. A small tube is placed through the cervix into the uterus and connected to a vacuum machine. This removes any tissue remaining in the uterus. It serves the same function as a D&C but is usually preferred for an incomplete miscarriage because it is easier on an already-softened uterus, faster, more complete and less painful than a regular D&C.

61. *When is each procedure used?*

It depends on your doctor, where the procedure is performed and which method is preferred. If the procedure is done in the emergency room of a hospital, a suction-curettage machine is often available and is used because it gives a more-complete emptying of the uterus in shorter time.

62. *Is a suction curettage or D&C a painful procedure?*

Either procedure can cause some cramping while the uterus is being cleaned. It is usually no more painful than cramps you experience during the miscarriage.

63. *What determines if I need a D&C or suction curettage after a miscarriage?*

If the miscarriage is early, before the first 8 weeks after your last menstrual period, the uterine contents may be completely expelled from the uterus and nothing further will have to be done. This is called a *complete miscarriage.*

If the pregnancy has developed for more than 8 weeks, there's a greater chance all the tissue has not been expelled from the uterus. This is called an *incomplete miscarriage.* With an incomplete miscarriage, D&C or suction curettage is necessary.

64. *What are symptoms of an incomplete miscarriage?*

Persistent bleeding or cramping after a miscarriage are signs that tissue remains in the uterus. A D&C or suction curettage should be performed.

65. *What happens if a D&C or suction curettage is not performed?*

Retained tissue could lead to infection or development of scar tissue in the uterus or Fallopian tubes; this could cause problems with future fertility.

66. *Would I be put to sleep for a D&C or suction curettage?*

It depends on you, your doctor and your symptoms. Most of the time, either surgery can be performed in a doctor's office or an emergency room, if equipment is available, without general anesthesia.

67. *Can anything be done to lessen the pain?*

A paracervical block into the cervix can lessen pain and cramps. In most cases, the procedure takes about 5 minutes.

68. *What if I am apprehensive or fearful of pain?*

If you are very apprehensive or fearful, it is possible to give you a general anesthetic in the operating room.

69. *What is a habitual miscarriage?*

Three or more consecutive miscarriages is called *habitual* or *repeated miscarriage*.

70. *What causes habitual miscarriage?*

There are many reasons for habitual miscarriage, and they are divided into five categories—genetic (chromosomal), infectious, hormonal, anatomical and environmental.

71. *What are genetic causes?*

If you have three or more miscarriages in a row, there is a 10% chance you or your husband have a chromosome abnormality. Chromosomes are rod-shaped structures that appear in all our body cells. The genes they contain are the hereditary messages passed on to the baby.

72. *How many chromosomes do we have?*

Each of us has 22 pairs of chromosomes, called *autosomes*, and one pair of sex chromosomes. A woman has two X sex chromosomes, and a man has one X and one Y sex chromosome. A woman is referred to as XX and a man as XY.

The fertilized egg gets half its chromosomes from the mother and half from the father, but the *sperm* determines the sex of a child. An egg always contains an X chromosome. The sperm passes either an X or Y chromosome to the egg when fertilization occurs. If an X chromosome is passed, the baby is a girl. If the Y chromosome is passed, the baby is a boy because the Y chromosome is dominant.

73. *How can an abnormal chromosome cause a miscarriage?*

One of you may carry a chromosome or part of a chromosome that is not lined up in the proper order. This misalignment, called *translocation*, could be passed on to the fertilized egg. This is not compatible with a developing fetus, and a miscarriage occurs.

74. *How can we make sure our chromosomes are normal?*

A blood test, called *karyotyping*, can check your chromosomes. With habitual miscarriage, karyotyping should be done. It is expensive to do, so it is usually not done after a single miscarriage.

75. *Is there a treatment for abnormal chromosomes?*

No, there is not.

76. *If there's no treatment, why do the test?*

So you'll know exactly what your problem is instead of relying on false hope. Genetic counseling can give you the odds of having another miscarriage or a normal pregnancy.

77. *Is it possible for us to have a normal pregnancy under these circumstances?*

Often, even with repeated miscarriages with a chromosomal abnormality, you may eventually have a normal pregnancy.

78. *Can infection cause miscarriages?*

Various infections during the first several months of pregnancy that cause a fever of 103 to 104F (39 to 40C) may affect a developing pregnancy and cause miscarriage. A viral illness, such as rubella, during pregnancy can affect a developing fetus. Rubella can cause miscarriage and birth defects in a fetus. Women with autoimmune disorders, such as lupus erythematosis, and women with diabetes have a higher incidence of miscarriages and birth defects.

79. *Can infections of my cervix and vagina cause miscarriages?*

Various infections caused by chlamydia, mycoplasma and B-streptococcus can interfere with fertility and may cause early miscarriage.

80. *How can these infections be detected?*

Cultures can be done by your doctor to detect the organisms.

81. *How are these infections treated?*

If any of these organisms is present, antibiotics can be prescribed.

82. *Is there a risk in taking antibiotics during pregnancy?*

Certain antibiotics are safe to take during pregnancy, but other antibiotics should be avoided. Your doctor will know the appropriate antibiotic to prescribe.

83. *What are the hormonal factors that play a part in miscarriage?*

A condition called *luteal phase defect*, which may play a part in becoming pregnant, can also play a part in causing an early miscarriage.

84. *What is a luteal phase defect?*

After you ovulate, the area in the ovary that expelled the egg changes to a corpus luteum. A corpus luteum secretes progesterone until the placenta of a developing pregnancy is large enough to take over production. Progesterone is needed to change the lining of the uterus to support the implanted pregnancy.

85. *What if there is not enough progesterone?*

If there isn't enough progesterone present, the pregnancy will not be supported, and a miscarriage will occur.

86. *How is luteal phase defect diagnosed?*

Your doctor can compare your basal body temperatures with an endometrial biopsy to see if they are "in phase" with each other.

The purpose of performing an endometrial biopsy is to document ovulation and determine where you are in your menstrual cycle. The pathologist who reads your biopsy determines this by examining the biopsy and comparing the way the endometrial cells and tissue surrounding the cells appear.

A gynecologic-pathologist can look at the uterine lining and determine within a few days where you are in your cycle. This determination is compared to your BBT taken that month and the time you actually start your period. If these all correspond within 2 days, it is normal. If there is a big discrepancy, it is called "being out of phase."

87. *How is luteal phase defect treated?*

It can be treated with the fertility drug clomiphene citrate, HCG or progesterone given in the form of a vaginal suppository.

88. *What if pregnancy occurs when a luteal phase defect is present?*

If pregnancy occurs, it may be helpful to continue to use progesterone suppositories until the placenta is fully developed (until about the third month of pregnancy). This gives the pregnancy the added progesterone to support the uterine lining until the placenta takes over production of progesterone.

89. *Can disorders of other endocrine glands cause miscarriages?*

Disorders of the thyroid gland, adrenal gland or pancreas may occasionally cause a miscarriage.

90. *What anatomical factors can cause a miscarriage?*

Malformations of the uterus, such as a septum (a dividing wall or partition within the uterine cavity), double uterus or a T-shaped uterus may cause you to miscarry. See illustrations on pages 98 and 99.

Adhesions inside the uterus, called *Asherman's Syndrome,* an incompetent cervix and uterine myomas can also cause miscarriages. Some of these conditions may cause a premature delivery between 20 and 30 weeks of pregnancy, rather than a miscarriage (pregnancy loss before the 20th week).

91. *How are anatomical abnormalities detected?*

They are usually found by performing a hysterogram (HSG). A pelvic examination performed by your doctor may also detect abnormalities.

92. *How can anatomical abnormalities of the uterus be treated?*

Surgery is usually necessary to correct a septum or fibroid tumor.

93. *How is a double uterus treated?*

A double uterus may not be correctable, but there are several variations to this condition. Some are more serious than others. Your doctor or any specialist you are referred to will decide a course of action. When you have a double uterus, often each pregnancy continues longer, hopefully to produce a living baby.

94. *How is Asherman's Syndrome treated?*

Asherman's Syndrome is treated in one of three ways:
● With a D&C or hysteroscopy to cut the adhesions present in the uterine cavity.
● By placing an IUD in the uterus to keep adhesions from forming again.
● Treatment with estrogen to stimulate the endometrium to grow.

95. *What is an incompetent cervix?*

A normal cervix dilates only in labor so the baby can come out. In some cases, the cervix is unable to hold the contents of the developing pregnancy and prematurely opens between 20 and 36 weeks of pregnancy. If delivery is too early, a premature baby may be born, with little chance of surviving.

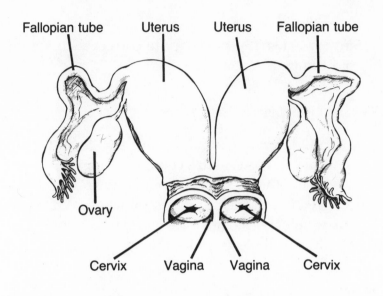

Fallopian tube   Uterus   Uterus   Fallopian tube

Ovary

Cervix   Vagina   Vagina   Cervix

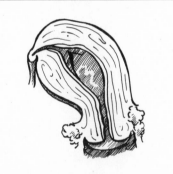

Above:
Double uterus with double cervix and double vagina.

Left:
Uterus with uterine horn and one Fallopian tube.

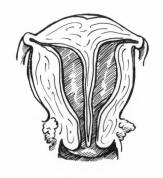
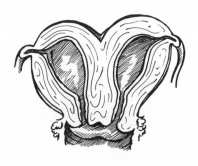
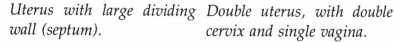

Uterus with large dividing wall (septum).

Double uterus, with double cervix and single vagina.

96. *What causes an incompetent cervix?*

There are several possible causes of an incompetent cervix. Women whose mothers took DES while they were pregnant with them have a greater chance of having an incompetent cervix. A cervical tear from a previous traumatic delivery may cause an incompetent cervix. Repeated forceful dilatations of the cervix from abortions may also be a factor. Some women are born with a congenital weakening of the cervix that results in an incompetent cervix.

97. *How can an incompetent cervix be treated?*

At between 14 and 20 weeks of pregnancy, a stitch can be placed around the cervix to help prevent it from prematurely opening. This procedure is called *cervical cerclage*. Medication to help relax the uterus, limited activity and bed rest may also be helpful.

98. *How are uterine myomas treated?*

If your doctor feels they are contributing to your infertility, a myomectomy should be performed. See page 143.

99. *Can exposure to drugs, chemicals and other substances cause miscarriages?*

Exposure to potent drugs, such as LSD, drugs used to treat cancer and excessive X-ray exposure to the fetus may play a factor in miscarriages.

100. *What about medications?*

Over-the-counter medications and drugs normally prescribed by your physician do not cause miscarriages. But avoid them if you're pregnant until you discuss it with your doctor.

101. *Can occupational hazards increase my chances of miscarrying?*

Exposure to certain chemicals or pollutants in the workplace may cause you to miscarry. Exposure to anesthetic gases, lead and mercury poisoning, and exposure to chemicals, such as carbon disulfide, chloroprene and polychlorinated biphenyls (PCB), have all been associated with increased miscarriage rates.

102. *How long after a miscarriage should we wait to try to become pregnant again?*

Most doctors advise you to have two or three normal periods before trying to become pregnant. This allows the uterine lining a chance to return to normal.

103. *Should birth control be used during that time?*

A barrier method of birth control (foam, condoms, diaphragm) is the most useful method of contraception for this short interval.

104. *Is it normal to become depressed after experiencing a miscarriage?*

Yes, it's normal to feel upset and depressed, especially if you have a history of infertility. But if you have been infertile, having a miscarriage is often a good sign—it shows you're capable of becoming pregnant. Hopefully, the next time you become pregnant it will be successful.

105. *Is it common for me to blame myself for a miscarriage?*

After a miscarriage you may review your activity to try to find a reason or blame yourself for the miscarriage. Some women view their miscarriage as a form of punishment.

No one's to blame—not yourself, your husband or your doctor. Healthy pregnancies have remained intact after horseback riding, skiing, heavy lifting and strenuous activities. It isn't your fault if you miscarry.

106. *Do couples become distant following a miscarriage?*

Occasionally this happens. This may be due to the grieving both go through. If this happens to you, it's important to discuss your feelings and frustrations with each other. Keep communication open.

107. *Are some couples afraid to have sexual intercourse after a miscarriage?*

Your doctor may recommend you avoid intercourse for 10 to 14 days after a miscarriage. Occasionally, you may be afraid to have intercourse from fear of becoming pregnant and having another miscarriage.

108. *What should be done about lingering emotional trauma following a miscarriage?*

Talk with your doctor. If he feels you might benefit from further counseling, he'll refer you to someone who has experience in dealing with this problem. There are also support groups in many cities that can help. Often discussing the problem with someone who has gone through the same emotional trauma can help.

5

How Is Infertility in a Woman Diagnosed?

When you suspect you and your husband may have a fertility problem, you are probably the one to begin asking questions and seeking answers. This section is devoted to infertility problems in women, and the questions and answers relate directly to diagnosis and prognosis of the situation. The causes and treatments of infertility in women are covered in the next section, which begins on page 125. Diagnosis, causes and treatments of infertility in men are discussed in following sections.

1. *When should I go to my doctor for help?*

Although infertility is defined as "not being able to conceive after 1 year of trying," some women seek help before a year is up. There is no set time interval when you should go to your doctor. If you're over 30 years old, you may want to seek help earlier than a woman in her early 20s. If you're becoming frustrated from not conceiving, see your doctor for an exam and preliminary tests.

2. *How expensive is an infertility examination?*

It depends on what has to be done. The initial interview and exam may be in the range of $45 to $75. Often this is all that is required. If a full "work up" is needed, it usually costs several hundred dollars. If surgery and hospitalization are also needed, it may cost several thousand dollars.

3. *Does medical insurance pay for an infertility investigation?*

It depends on the type of medical insurance you have.

4. *How long does an infertility work up take?*

Most basic tests can be completed in 4 to 8 weeks. Occasionally, tests must be repeated if they are not normal or do not correspond with the results of other tests.

5. *How often will I need to visit my doctor during an infertility work up?*

It depends on the number of tests the doctor feels are necessary. The timing of the tests is usually scheduled according to your menstrual cycle. Most of an infertility work up can be completed in two menstrual cycles.

6. *Are infertility tests painful?*

It depends on you and the tests performed. One test involves only a pelvic examination (post-coital test). Other tests, such as a hysterosalpingogram (X-ray of the tubes and uterus), may cause menstrual-type cramps and low abdominal pain. If laparoscopy is needed, it may cause abdominal and chest discomfort.

For some women, infertility tests can be physically and emotionally strenuous. If testing becomes too strenuous, tests can be spread out over a longer period of time. Some couples feel the sooner all tests are completed, the better they will feel because they will have the answers to their questions.

7. *What will tests for me involve?*

Tests for you include a pelvic examination after intercourse (post-coital test), recording your basal body temperature, an X-ray study of your uterus and possible minor surgery to look at internal organs.

8. *What will tests for my husband involve?*

The main test for a man is a semen analysis. If the semen analysis is normal, further testing is usually unnecessary. If the test is abnormal, further testing of the man is necessary.

9. *What can I expect on my first visit to the doctor?*

Your first visit will include a complete review of your past medical history including any tests you may already have had at another doctor's office. The doctor will make sure there are no general health problems accounting for your infertility. He will concentrate on your menstrual history and any problems you may have had with your periods or female organs. A complete physical exam, including a pelvic examination, will also be performed.

10. *Should my husband be present during the initial interview?*

It isn't necessary for your husband to be present, but it's important for him to be part of an infertility investigation. The doctor may have questions about your husband's health or job that you're unable to answer. It also helps prevent problems between you and your husband regarding evaluation and testing.

11. *What is included in my physical examination?*

The doctor will check your height, weight and blood pressure, and perform a general physical exam including heart, lung and breast examinations. He will pay special attention to abnormalities of your skin, such as excessive acne, and abnormal distributions of body hair and body fat.

12. *How does acne, body hair and body-fat distribution relate to infertility?*

It may indicate an excessive hormone production from the ovaries or adrenal glands. Excessive hormone production may prevent you from ovulating.

13. *What is a pelvic exam?*

It is an examination of your internal and external female organs. You disrobe below the waist, then lie down on an examination table. Your doctor places an instrument called a *speculum* into your vagina to open it so he can look directly at the vagina and cervix. A Pap smear is often done at this time; other cultures may also be done to check for possible infections.

After removing the speculum, the doctor places one hand in the vagina and one hand on the abdomen to feel for organ abnormalities.

14. *What is a Pap smear?*

It is a test to determine if abnormal cells are growing in the cervix. The test is done to detect cancer or precancerous conditions. The doctor scrapes cells off the surface of the cervix with a small spatula and places cells and secretions on a slide. This is sent to the lab to check for precancerous or cancerous cells.

15. *What other tests are done?*

Usually a blood test, called a *hemoglobin test,* is done to check the iron content of your blood. A urinalysis may be needed to see if you have an infection, protein or sugar in your urine.

16. *Will any other blood tests be done?*

It depends on your medical history and general physical exam. The doctor may want to repeat tests that were performed at another doctor's office. The following tests are often ordered as part of an infertility investigation to see if the appropriate organ or gland is functioning normally.

Blood Test	Organ Being Tested
Serum testosterone	Ovaries or adrenal gland
Dehydroepiandosterone sulfate (DHEAS)	Adrenal gland
Thyroid profile	Thyroid gland
Serum prolactin	Pituitary gland
Serum FSH & LH	Pituitary gland and ovary
Serum progesterone	Ovary

17. *Why are these tests important?*

They play an important role in an infertility investigation. Abnormalities of these organs and glands can lead to faulty sperm production in a man and ovulation disorders in a woman.

18. *Will the doctor do any other tests?*

There are four basic tests your doctor should perform during an infertility investigation:
- Basal body temperature
- Semen analysis
- Post-coital test
- Hysterosalpingogram

19. *What is the basal body temperature?*

It is a body temperature that helps determine if you are ovulating. See page 53. You take your basal (at rest) temperature before you get out of bed in the morning and record it daily on a graph. A normal basal-body-temperature graph reveals a lower temperature for the first part of the menstrual cycle. When ovulation occurs, the temperature rises and remains steady until menstruation occurs, at which time the temperature falls back to the preovulation range.

20. *Why does the temperature shift occur?*

The corpus luteum of the ovary secretes pro-gesterone after ovulation—the progesterone causes the temperature control center in the hypothalmus to raise the basal temperature.

21. *What if the temperature does not shift?*

It could mean you aren't ovulating.

22. *What is a semen analysis?*

Semen analysis is important in evaluating a couple's infertility. Your husband's semen and sperm are eval-uated for sperm count, sperm motility and other fac-tors. *Encourage your physician to do a semen analysis early in your fertility evaluation.* See pages 177 to 182.

23. *What is a post-coital test?*

Your doctor does a pelvic exam (within 12 hours) after you and your husband have intercourse. The test evaluates your cervical mucus and the number and motility of the sperm present in the mucus. This test determines if the cervical mucus and sperm are compatible with each other. In some cases, mucus prevents the sperm from staying alive while in the mucus. The post-coital test is also called a *Huhner's test.*

24. *Is there a certain time of the month when a post-coital test should be performed?*

Yes, it should be performed as close to ovulation time as possible. This is when cervical mucus is at its peak to accept sperm.

25. *How is a post-coital test performed?*

You and your husband have intercourse from 2 to 12 hours before you go to your doctor's office. The doctor performs a pelvic exam to obtain some of the cervical mucus. Mucus is placed on a slide, then examined under a microscope to see if any sperm are present. The doctor counts the number of sperm present, noting both active and inactive sperm.

26. *What is a normal post-coital-test result?*

Cervical mucus should be thin and stretchy; mucus is elastic or stretchy if it is at its peak. Many active (moving) sperm should be present in the mucus, with few inactive (non-moving or dead) sperm.

27. *What is considered an abnormal post-coital test?*

You have an abnormal test result if no sperm or very few sperm are present in the mucus or if many sperm are present, but none are moving.

28. *What causes an abnormal post-coital test?*

There can be many causes of an abnormal test. Abnormal cervical mucus consisting of too little mucus or "cloudy" mucus from an infection will kill sperm. An abnormal semen analysis, such as absent sperm, a very low sperm count or poor sperm motility, will cause an abnormal result.

Occasionally intercourse performed "on demand" for a test results in impotence or partial ejaculation with no sperm present. If the test is performed at a time you are not close to ovulation, mucus will be poor, with an abnormal result.

29. *How valuable is the post-coital test?*

It is possibly the single most important infertility test. If you have a normal test, it generally means your husband has a normal semen analysis. It shows your cervical mucus is adequate and your technique of intercourse is satisfactory. A normal post-coital test shows sperm and cervical mucus are compatible, and sperm stay alive in the mucus. Unfortunately, many doctors do not do this test early enough in an infertility evaluation.

30. *When should a post-coital test be done?*

The test should be one of the first tests performed as part of an infertility investigation. It should be done at the time of or a few days before ovulation. If you can schedule your first infertility visit at or close to ovulation time, you and your husband should have intercourse the night before or the morning of the appointment. Tell your doctor so he can perform this test on your first visit.

31. *What is a hysterosalpingogram?*

It is an X-ray study in which dye is injected through the cervix into the uterine cavity and out the Fallopian tubes. The test indicates abnormalities of the uterine cavity and determines whether Fallopian tubes are open. The test is often called a *hysterogram* or *HSG*.

32. *Where is the test performed?*

Your doctor can usually perform this test in the X-ray department of a hospital. If his office has X-ray equipment, he may perform the test there.

33. *Is the test painful?*

Some women have moderately severe cramps similar to menstrual cramps; others feel little pain.

34. *Is an anesthetic given?*

Usually not, although if you have severe menstrual

cramps, you may be more sensitive to pain in the pelvis. You may benefit from a paracervical block.

35. *What is a paracervical block?*

It is an injection of an anesthetic into the cervix. It numbs the cervix to lessen cramps.

36. *Will the doctor require assistance while performing HSG?*

Yes. A technician will assist the doctor and take the X-rays; a radiologist will read the X-rays.

37. *How is the test performed?*

A speculum is placed into your vagina, then the doctor places an instrument (a hysterogram canula) into your cervical canal. A radio-opaque dye, which can be seen on an X-ray, is injected into your uterus and tubes. The dye can be seen on a monitor as it goes into the uterine cavity.

38. *Are there any risks in having this test?*

A hysterosalpingogram exposes you to a small dose of radiation, but the exposure is low so benefits from the test outweigh the amount of radiation you receive. There is also a very small risk of developing a uterine or tubal infection following the procedure.

39. *At what point in my menstrual cycle is this test performed?*

It should be performed after you stop menstruating but before ovulation occurs, usually between day 7 and day 12 of your cycle. This eliminates radiation exposure and injecting dye into a uterus where a pregnancy may be developing.

40. *How long does it take to get the results of the test?*

In most cases results are known immediately. Sometimes a more detailed study of the X-rays must be made before a conclusion can be reached.

41. *What if the findings are inconclusive or there is a suspicion of blocked tubes?*

Further investigation may be necessary. Your doctor will usually suggest a laparoscopy examination. See page 119.

42. *Can blocked tubes be opened by a hysterosalpingogram?*

It's possible very small, filmy adhesions can be broken by the pressure of the dye going through the tubes. Many women have become pregnant following a hysterosalpingogram. Whether it has cured small, filmy adhesions or it was coincidental is unknown.

43. *Are there other tests to determine if Fallopian tubes are open?*

A laparoscopy examination and a test called the

Rubin test can be performed to determine if tubes are blocked or open.

44. *What is the Rubin test?*

This test was more frequently performed in the past. Carbon dioxide gas is injected through the cervix into the uterus, similar to the way dye is injected in a hysterosalpingogram. The gas goes into the uterus and makes its way out the Fallopian tubes. The gas then goes into the abdominal cavity and under the diaphragm where it causes pain in the shoulder. Shoulder pain is the test result we are looking for. If pain is present, it usually means at least one tube is open.

45. *Why isn't a Rubin test performed as often today?*

This test doesn't provide as much information as HSG. If you have pain in the shoulders from the Rubin test, it's impossible to tell if one or both tubes are open. A hysterosalpingogram also tells if your uterine cavity and both Fallopian tubes are normal.

46. *When would a doctor choose a Rubin test instead of doing a hysterosalpingogram?*

The Rubin test may be performed if you are allergic to radio-opaque dyes. It also can be performed in the doctor's office, without X-ray equipment, and may be useful as a quick screening test.

47. *What other tests, besides the BBT, can be performed to see if I am ovulating?*

Other tests for ovulation include endometrial biopsy, serum progesterone, ultrasound of the ovaries or directly looking at the ovaries with laparoscopy. The recently developed ovulation predictor tests, such as OvuStick, First Response and OvuTime, can also be used. See pages 61 to 63.

48. *What is an endometrial biopsy?*

It is a sampling of the tissue of the uterine lining (endometrium).

49. *Where is the test performed?*

It is performed in the doctor's office.

50. *When is the best time to do an endometrial biopsy?*

It's best to do an endometrial biopsy after suspected ovulation, usually a few days before your expected period. Results of the biopsy are compared with the basal-body-temperature graph to make sure they are in phase with each other.

51. *What does it mean to be "in phase"?*

To be *in phase* means the reading on the endometrial biopsy is at about the same day as you are in your menstrual cycle.

52. *How is an endometrial biopsy performed?*

Your doctor inserts a small tube through the cervix into your uterine cavity. He withdraws the tube, trapping a small piece of tissue in it. Tissue is sent to a pathologist to be examined under a microscope to see if ovulation has occurred and to "date" the endometrium.

53. *What is dating the endometrium?*

The pathologist looks at the endometrial biopsy under the microscope and determines where you are in your menstrual cycle. A pathologist does this by looking for changes in the glands of the uterine lining and noting how compact the tissue is around the glands. This is important because it may indicate a luteal phase defect—the last half of the cycle is short. An endometrial biopsy may also show you are not ovulating at all, despite regular menstrual periods.

54. *What is a serum-progesterone test?*

It is a test to determine the level of progesterone in your blood. The progesterone level goes up after ovulation. Test results can be compared with normal progesterone levels before and after ovulation.

55. *What is ultrasound?*

Ultrasound uses sound waves instead of X-rays to project a picture on a monitor. Your doctor can look directly at the inside of your abdominal and pelvic cavity to see the ovaries and determine if a developing egg is present.

56. *How is ultrasound used in an infertility investigation?*

It can determine if ovulation is about to occur—this is a new, sophisticated way of seeing how your ovaries swell just before ovulation then become smaller after ovulation.

Ultrasound is becoming popular in timing ovulation before artificial insemination, in conjunction with Pergonal administration and in-vitro fertilization. Ultrasound visualization of the ovaries is usually unnecessary for routine infertility investigation.

57. *What is laparoscopy?*

Laparoscopy is a minor surgical procedure that involves placing a laparoscope through the navel to look directly at abdominal and pelvic organs. It involves minor surgery, so it is often a final diagnostic procedure in an infertility work up.

Laparoscopy can be performed with one incision or with two incisions. Most doctors use the two-incision method—one incision is made in the navel for the laparoscope and another incision is made in the pubic hairline for the instruments, such as scissors, cautery and probe attachment. With the operating instruments away from the laparoscope, the surgeon can see better and has greater mobility in performing surgical procedures. See illustration on opposite page.

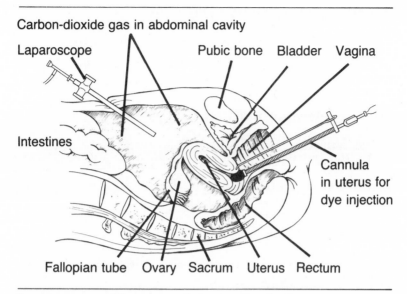

Carbon-dioxide gas in abdominal cavity

Laparoscope　　　　　　　　Pubic bone　Bladder　Vagina

Intestines

Cannula
in uterus for
dye injection

Fallopian tube　Ovary　Sacrum　Uterus　Rectum

Laparoscopy with woman lying on her back.

58. *What is the purpose of a laparoscopy exam?*

There are several reasons to do a laparoscopy with an infertility work up. If the results of the hysterosalpingogram are inconclusive or show blocked tubes, looking directly at the tubes can determine how badly diseased the tubes are and what can be done to correct them. Scar tissue from past infections, surgery or endometriosis are visible.

Blue dye can be injected through the cervix and into the uterus during laparoscopy to see if Fallopian tubes are open. Another reason to perform laparoscopy is to see if endometriosis is present. Endometriosis is an important condition associated with infertility and is commonly found during laparoscopy. See the chapter on endometriosis, which begins on page 165.

59. *Where is a laparoscopy performed?*

It is usually performed in a hospital operating room or a surgical center under general anesthesia.

60. *Do I have to stay overnight in the hospital?*

No, you don't. Usually you go into the hospital in the morning, have the procedure done and go home a few hours later after effects of the anesthetic wear off.

61. *How is laparoscopy performed?*

After you are asleep on the operating table, you are put into a position similar to having a pelvic exam. Instruments are placed in the cervix so the uterus can be manipulated and dye can be injected during the procedure. Instruments placed on the cervix are similar to those used during a hysterosalpingogram.

An incision is made through the navel, and a special needle is inserted into the abdominal cavity. Carbon dioxide gas is pumped into the abdominal cavity to push abdominal muscles away from the intestines to create space for the laparoscope.

In some cases, a second, smaller, incision is made at the level of the pubic hairline. This allows instruments to be placed through the laparoscope for operating and manipulating the uterus, tubes or ovaries.

62. *What types of minor surgery can be performed through a laparoscope?*

Small adhesions can be cut, endometriosis implants can be cauterized and fluid can be withdrawn from ovarian cysts. Occasionally, a tubal or ectopic pregnancy can be removed with laparoscopy. If a woman wants to be sterilized, the tubes can be cauterized or clips can be placed on them.

63. *Is laparoscopy used for purposes other than infertility?*

Yes, it is. Laparoscopy is used to evaluate unexplained pelvic pain and in cases of suspected appendicitis or ectopic pregnancy.

The procedure is also used by other surgeons to diagnose abdominal conditions, especially liver diseases. Laparoscopy is also the most common way women elect to have permanent sterilization performed.

64. *Is laparoscopy painful?*

You are given general anesthesia when a laparoscopy is performed, so you don't feel pain during the procedure. The amount of discomfort afterward varies. There may be shoulder and chest discomfort from gas pumped into the abdominal cavity during the procedure. There may also be abdominal discomfort around the incisions. Most women can usually resume normal activities in 1 or 2 days.

65. *Is it possible for me to see what my doctor sees in my pelvis during laparoscopy?*

Some physicians now record all their laparoscopy findings on videocassette and show them to their patients after the procedure. This has been made possible by a recently developed video camera that fits over the laparoscope. Recording the procedure has been useful to physicians in helping explain laparoscopy findings to their patients.

66. What is culdoscopy?

A culdoscope is an instrument similar to the laparoscope; it uses a fiberoptic light source for illumination and examination. The culdoscope is different because it gives a right-angle view to the direction of the scope—laparoscopy is usually a direct projection.

In culdoscopy, the instrument is placed through the culdesac, the area at the top of the vagina behind the cervix, to look directly at the uterus, tubes and ovaries. Culdoscopy only allows examination of the posterior part of the uterus; complete examination of the ovaries is not always possible. See illustration on opposite page.

67. Why is culdoscopy not performed much today?

The laparoscope has replaced the culdoscope because laparoscopy gives a more complete view of the pelvis and abdomen and allows more room to maneuver and operate.

68. What is hysteroscopy?

Hysteroscopy is another procedure that uses a fiberoptic-light source; it is used to look directly inside the uterine cavity.

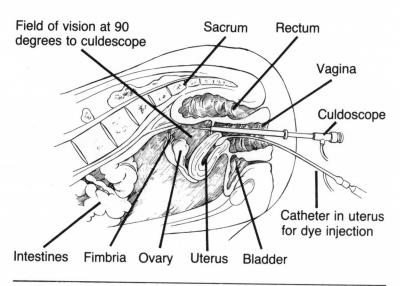

Culdoscopy with woman lying on her abdomen.

69. *What purpose does a hysteroscopy have in an infertility investigation?*

If a suspicious bump or adhesion is seen inside the uterus on a hysterosalpingogram, the hysteroscope can be inserted into the uterine cavity to examine the abnormality. If Asherman's Syndrome is discovered, the hysteroscope is used to cut the adhesions or a hysterosalpingogram, see illustration on page 124, can be performed. If a polyp is present, it can be removed with a hysteroscope.

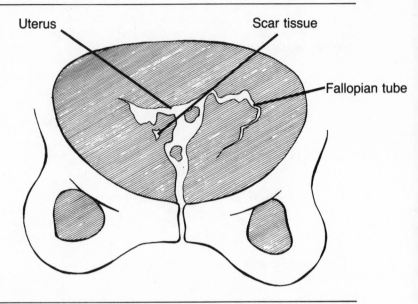

Hysterogram (hysterosalpingogram) view of Asherman's Syndrome showing scar tissue in the uterus.

70. *Where is a hysteroscopy procedure performed?*

It can be done in your doctor's office with a local anesthetic but is more commonly done in the hospital. Often a hysteroscopy exam is performed at the same time as laparoscopy.

6

What Are the Causes and Treatments of Infertility in a Woman?

Many times, a woman will become pregnant by the time her basic fertility evaluation is completed. Some reasons for infertility are simple, such as timing of intercourse, using vaginal lubricants or other reasons that are discussed at the first visit. Other reasons are much more complicated.

There are many causes of female infertility. Researchers appear to be discovering new causes of infertility every year.

1. *What is the most common cause of infertility in a woman?*

This is difficult to answer because there are so *many* different causes of infertility. The most common cause (for about 50% of the cases) is failure to ovulate— either total failure to ovulate or failure to ovulate regularly. This is usually caused by the complex hormonal regulation of the ovaries by the hypothalmus and pituitary glands. Often, failure to ovulate may be associated with other causes of infertility.

The causes of infertility are usually broken down into major groups, which include:

- Vaginal factors
- Cervical factors
- Uterine factors
- Tubal factors
- Ovarian factors

2. *How is an ovulation problem in a woman detected?*

Failure to ovulate is usually suspected if you have irregular periods or go several months without a period. Infertility investigation tests—BBT and endometrial biopsy—are used to determine if you are ovulating.

3. *Is an ovulation problem easily corrected?*

Most cases of ovulation disorders are correctable with ovulation-inducing drugs, such as clomiphene citrate. Other cases can be very resistant to medication, and other remedies may be needed, including using Pergonal, combining clomiphene citrate with HCG, or using GNRH and bromocryptine.

4. *What are other causes of infertility in a woman?*

The second major cause of infertility in a woman is tubal disease, which accounts for 33% of all cases of female infertility. Adhesions, partial blockage or total blockage of the Fallopian tubes prevent the egg and sperm from uniting.

In addition to ovarian disease and tubal disease, uterine factors, cervical factors, endometriosis and sperm "allergy" can attribute to your infertility.

5. *How are these problems detected?*

Tubal disease is usually detected when HSG or laparoscopy is performed. Other causes are usually detected as part of the routine investigation—post-coital tests, hysterogram and a pelvic exam.

6. *Are these problems easily correctable?*

Tubal disease is not as easily treated as ovulation disorders in most cases. Surgery is usually required—either laparoscopy or major abdominal surgery—to correct tubal disease. Success in treating tubal disease is usually not as good as treating ovulation disorders.

VAGINAL FACTORS

7. *What is a vaginal factor in infertility?*

For you to become pregnant, sperm must be able to get into the vagina by an appropriate intercourse technique. Occasionally this is not possible. For lack of a better term, we have decided to call a group of conditions "vaginal factors"—these factors prevent sperm from entering the vagina or sperm that does enter the vagina can't enter the cervical mucus.

An example of a vaginal factor would be a couple that is so obese that the penis cannot enter the vagina. Vaginal factors also include vaginal infections, which may interfere with sperm survival.

8. *What is an "appropriate intercourse technique"?*

An appropriate intercourse technique is any method of intercourse in which sperm get into the vagina and cervical mucus. This includes *not* using artificial lubricants that may kill sperm and *not* getting up to go to the bathroom or to douche immediately after intercourse.

9. *How is marked obesity in a couple treated if they wish to become pregnant?*

If normal intercourse positions do not allow sperm to enter the vagina, and the problem can't be corrected by changing positions, artificial insemination may be necessary to achieve pregnancy.

10. *Can lack of lubrication during intercourse be a problem in achieving pregnancy?*

Lack of lubrication can make intercourse difficult. This problem is often caused by inadequate sexual foreplay before intercourse. When intercourse is done "on demand," it's easy to forget that adequate foreplay is necessary to achieve lubrication in a woman.

11. *Should artificial lubrication by used?*

No. Artificial lubricants, such as petroleum jelly or K-Y jelly, should not be used because they may kill sperm.

12. *Should I lie down following intercourse?*

Yes. Lie on your back or side for 15 to 20 minutes following intercourse to keep sperm from leaking out of the vagina. Don't get up to urinate or douche.

13. *Can vaginal infections cause infertility?*

Possibly, especially if they are severe. The vagina and cervix are in close proximity to each other—a vaginal infection may also involve the cervical mucus and interfere with sperm survival and motility.

There are three main types of vaginal infections called *vaginitis*. These include yeast infections, trichomonas and gardnerella infections. If these infections are left untreated, they may affect your ability to become pregnant or cause excessive vaginal and external genital irritation and make intercourse uncomfortable.

14. *What is a yeast infection?*

A yeast infection is a vaginal infection caused by a fungus. It is common in women who take antibiotics and birth-control pills, women with diabetes and women who are pregnant. It is also common during hot, humid weather and in women who perspire a lot, such as women runners.

15. *What are symptoms of a yeast infection?*

A white, cheesy, vaginal discharge and severe itching and burning in the vagina and external genital area are the most common symptoms.

16. *What is trichomonas?*

Trichomonas is a vaginal infection caused by a protozoa called *trichomonas vaginalis.*

17. *What are the symptoms of a trichomonas infection?*

A very red, inflamed vagina and cervix, a foul-smelling discharge and external genital irritation are common symptoms.

18. *What is a gardnerella infection?*

Gardnerella is a vaginal infection caused by bacteria; it results in a light-green discharge with a "fishy" odor. Gardnerella infections are also called *hemophilus* or *non-specific vaginal infections.*

19. *How are vaginal infections diagnosed?*

They are diagnosed by doing a pelvic exam, then examining vaginal secretions under a microscope. Each organism—yeast, trichomanas and gardnerella—has a typical look when examined under a microscope, and they can usually be easily diagnosed.

20. *How are vaginal infections treated?*

Treatment for each infection is different and usually consists of using a vaginal cream or suppository for a yeast infection and an antibiotic for the other infections.

21. *Are both partners treated?*

It is not necessary to treat both partners when a yeast infection is present. It is best to treat both if a trichomonas or gardnerella infection is present.

22. *Should I try to become pregnant if I have a vaginal infection?*

It is not harmful to have intercourse to try to conceive during this time. It may be uncomfortable if the infection causes vaginal and genital irritation.

CERVICAL FACTORS

23. *I've heard problems with my cervix and cervical mucus can cause infertility. Can you explain this?*

The cervix is the point where sperm leave the vagina to make their way toward the egg in the Fallopian tube. Because the pH of the vagina is very acid, sperm cannot live long in the vagina. They must get into the cervical mucus, which is very alkaline and compatible with sperm survival. If cervical mucus is not present, if it is cloudy and thick or if it contains antibodies that kill sperm, infertility will result.

Cervical factors or disorders of the cervix and cervical mucus account for about 10 to 15% of all cases of female infertility.

24. *What is the purpose of the cervix in fertility?*

The cervix secretes a watery mucus that begins to increase shortly after your period. It reaches its peak at the time of ovulation. If mucus is normal, it can be grasped between your fingers at the time of ovulation and stretched for several inches. The elasticity of the cervical mucus is called *spinnbarkeit*.

Cervical mucus is alkaline, as compared to the acid pH of the vagina. Sperm need an alkaline environment to survive.

25. *Why should mucus be thin and watery?*

This makes it easy for sperm to get into the uterus and Fallopian tubes.

26. *What happens to the mucus after ovulation?*

After ovulation, mucus becomes thick and cloudy. After your menstrual period, the cycle repeats itself going from thin, watery mucus to thick, cloudy mucus.

This change in cervical mucus can help predict your "fertile" time so you can time intercourse to become pregnant or avoid pregnancy.

27. *What abnormalities of the mucus can occur?*

There may be an inadequate amount of mucus, mucus may be too thick, or mucus may be "hostile" to sperm.

28. *How are mucus problems detected?*

Your doctor will detect problems with the mucus when he performs a post-coital test. See page 110.

29. *What causes an inadequate amount of mucus?*

Too little mucus can be caused by an inadequate amount of estrogen stimulation to the cervix or from previous surgery on the cervix resulting in fewer cervical glands.

30. *What is the treatment when there is not enough cervical mucus?*

If your doctor finds mucus is inadequate and there is no evidence of infection, he may give you a low-dose estrogen pill to stimulate the cervix to produce more mucus.

31. *Can previous surgery on the cervix affect fertility?*

Previous surgery on the cervix, such as conization, may remove most of the cervical glands or scar the cervix. Cauterization of the cervix may cause the same problem. Previous conization may also result in an incompetent cervix that cannot contain a pregnancy.

32. *What can be done to correct this problem?*

Low-dose estrogen and dilating the cervix many help. If they do not, intrauterine artificial insemination may be necessary to bypass cervical mucus.

33. *When is estrogen taken?*

It is taken before ovulation—during the first 10 to 14 days of your menstrual cycle—to avoid taking it in the event pregnancy occurs.

34. *What causes mucus to become too thick?*

This can result from various infections that cause an inflammation of the cervical glands, which produces a yellow or green discharge from the cervix. Some women normally secrete thick mucus.

35. *How can thick mucus be treated?*

If it is caused by infection, the infection is treated. If mucus is clear but thick, Robitussin (a cough medicine) may be taken orally to thin it. Robitussin contains a substance that breaks up thick secretions and has been found to be helpful in some cases of thick mucus. If this doesn't work, artificial insemination may be tried.

36. *What are the most common cervical infections?*

The most common cervical infections are gonorrhea, ureaplasma, mycoplasma and chlamydia.

37. *What are the symptoms of a cervical infection?*

A cervical infection may cause a vaginal discharge that stains your underwear. A mild infection may go undetected and not cause any symptoms.

In some cases, a cervical infection progresses into a uterine or tubal infection, causing symptoms of a generalized pelvic infection—low abdominal pain, cramps and fever.

38. *How do cervical infections contribute to infertility?*

Any cervical infection may affect the sperm's ability to survive in the mucus as it makes its way to meet the egg. Even a mild infection can affect fertility.

39. *How are these infections diagnosed?*

They are diagnosed by taking a culture from the cervix during a pelvic examination.

40. *What is a culture?*

A sample is taken of your cervical or vaginal secretions and sent to the laboratory to grow bacteria that causes the infection.

41. *How are these infections treated?*

Antibiotics, such as penicillin, ampicillin or tetracycline, usually cure these infections.

42. *Are both partners treated?*

Often both partners are treated, even if only one of them has an infection.

43. *Can a cervical infection cause other pelvic infections?*

If a cervical infection becomes severe or is left untreated, it is possible for it to progress to the uterus and Fallopian tubes. This may result in permanent scarring and possible blockage of Fallopian tubes.

44. *How can a person get these infections?*

They are transmitted by sexual intercourse.

45. *Does this mean a sexual partner passes on the infection?*

Not necessarily. Bacteria can be harbored deep in the cervical glands or the prostate gland. For reasons not completely understood, bacteria can suddenly cause an infection after being latent for some time. A person may have a low-grade infection for many years, without symptoms. Bacteria may be found when a culture is done as part of a routine fertility investigation.

46. *What is hostile mucus?*

It is a term used to describe sperm's inability to survive or immobilization of sperm, despite having clear mucus with excellent spinnbarkeit.

47. *What causes hostile mucus?*

Most cases of hostile cervical mucus are caused by an incompatibility between the mucus and sperm. It can be considered an allergy to sperm when sperm comes in contact with the mucus and they become immobilized.

48. *How is hostile mucus diagnosed?*

A post-coital test reveals dead sperm or very poorly moving sperm in the mucus. If this is found, the post-coital test should be repeated and further investigation may be necessary.

49. *Are there other abnormalities of the cervix that can cause infertility?*

Yes. Women who were exposed to DES often have an abnormal cervix. We now know many of these women have a higher incidence of infertility and miscarriage. The exact reasons for this are unknown.

Cervical factors, uterine factors and tubal factors may all be responsible.

50. *Is it possible for the cervix to be so tight that sperm can't get into the uterus?*

There is a difference of opinion on this. Most doctors feel if you are able to menstruate and blood can get out of the uterus, sperm can get in.

51. *What can be done about a tight cervix?*

The cervix can be gradually stretched with dilators placed through the cervical opening.

UTERINE FACTORS

52. *Can abnormalities of the uterus affect fertility?*

Yes. Infections, fibroid tumors and congenital abnormalities are uterine factors that affect fertility.

53. *What are infections of the uterus called?*

When you get an infection of the uterus, it is the *uterine lining* that becomes infected, not the muscle or body of the uterus. Infections of the uterus are really infections of the uterine lining (endometrium); that's why it is called *endometritis*.

54. *How does this infection occur?*

Endometritis can occur after having a baby, after an abortion or after a miscarriage. Endometritis is also associated with infections from an IUD. The uterine lining can also become inflamed when you have a generalized pelvic infection.

PID (pelvic inflammatory disease) is a general term that means inflammation of the pelvic organs including ovaries, tubes, uterus and cervix. PID can be caused by one of many organisms, such as gonorrhea, chlamydia and several other kinds of bacteria. It is not a specific disease but a term used for an entire *category* of diseases.

When you have PID, you probably have inflammation of your organs, including the ovary (oophoritis), Fallopian tubes (salpingitis), uterine lining (endometritis) and cervix (cervicitis).

Isolated infections of each organ are possible—you can have endometritis and not have salpingitis.

55. *How can endometritis interfere with fertility?*

During the acute phase of endometritis, the uterine lining is so inflamed that implantation cannot occur, so pregnancy is impossible. Once the infection heals, it is possible that scarring and adhesions form in the uterine cavity to close it off. This causes the walls of the uterus to "stick together." This results in very little, if any, endometrium in the uterine cavity.

If fertilization does occur, the fertilized egg cannot implant in the uterus. This condition is called *Asherman's Syndrome.*

56. *How is Asherman's Syndrome diagnosed?*

Symptoms include little or no bleeding at the time of your period because scarring has replaced your uterine lining. Your basal body temperature looks ovulatory because your ovaries still work despite a lack of periods. A hysterosalpingogram will show scarring in the uterus.

57. *What is the treatment for Asherman's Syndrome?*

Scarring and adhesions can be removed by D&C or hysteroscopy. Hysteroscopy is the preferred procedure because adhesions can be cut through the hysteroscope with scissors.

58. *What can be done to keep this condition from recurring?*

To prevent the uterus from scarring again, an IUD is placed in the uterine cavity to keep the walls separated. To stimulate the uterine lining to grow back, estrogen treatment is usually given for several months.

59. *Does estrogen always correct this condition?*

Occasionally scarring is so severe that estrogen will not rebuild the uterine lining. But about 70% of all women with Asherman's Syndrome eventually are able to conceive and carry a pregnancy to full term.

60. *When is the IUD removed?*

The IUD is left in for 3 to 6 months, until normal menstrual flow returns. A follow-up hysterogram helps determine if healing is complete.

61. *Are there any other treatments for this condition?*

There is no other known treatment for Asherman's Syndrome at this time.

62. *What are fibroids?*

Fibroids, also called *myomas,* are benign growths of the uterine muscle that can distort the uterine cavity.

63. *How do fibroids interfere with fertility?*

They may block the entrance into the uterus of the Fallopian tube. Fibroids may also prevent the fertilized egg from implanting in the uterine lining. See illustration on opposite page.

64. *Do all fibroids cause infertility?*

No. Many women conceive and have a normal pregnancy with fibroids present.

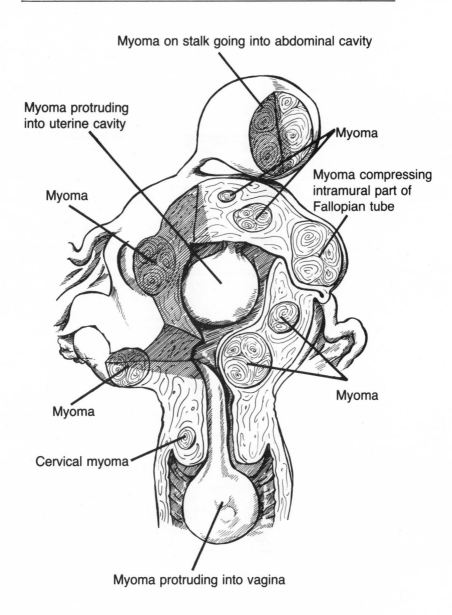

Myoma on stalk going into abdominal cavity

Myoma protruding
into uterine cavity

Myoma

Myoma

Myoma compressing
intramural part of
Fallopian tube

Myoma

Myoma

Cervical myoma

Myoma protruding into vagina

Cross section of uterus with myomas in the vagina and uterine cavity.

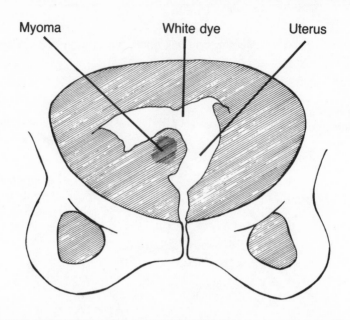

Myoma   White dye   Uterus

Hysterogram (hysterosalpingogram) view of myoma indenting the uterine cavity (white dye in the uterus).

65. *What other problems do fibroids cause?*

Fibroids may cause early miscarriages if they are located on the inner lining of the uterus. They may also block the birth canal and prevent a vaginal delivery.

If present during pregnancy, fibroids can grow rapidly and outgrow their blood supply. This causes acute abdominal pain.

66. *How are fibroids diagnosed?*

They can be felt during a pelvic examination, seen during a laparoscopy exam or seen on an X-ray when a hysterogram is done. See illustration above.

67. *How are fibroids treated?*

Surgery, called a *myomectomy*, is required to remove them, and it requires an abdominal incision. You spend 3 to 5 days in the hospital and are out of work 2 to 6 weeks. If fibroids are extensive, it may be impossible to remove them without removing the uterus; a hysterectomy may be necessary.

68. *What congenital abnormalities of the uterus can affect fertility?*

The uterus starts embryonic life as two separate systems that merge into one uterus. Failure of all or part of this system to merge can result in a double uterus with a double cervix, a double uterus with a single cervix, a single uterus with a dividing wall or a single cervix with two uterine horns (a small uterine cavity). See illustrations on pages 98 and 99.

69. *How do these abnormalities interfere with fertility?*

Abnormalities usually cause miscarriages and premature deliveries rather than preventing conception.

70. *What can be done about abnormalities?*

It depends on the severity of each condition. Often nothing can be done. If there is a septum in the uterus, it can be removed by surgery. This surgery is considered major surgery and is similar to a myomectomy. A small, thin septum is often removed through hysteroscopy.

TUBAL FACTORS

71. *What is the Fallopian tube's role in fertility?*

The Fallopian tube is a very important part of the female reproductive system. The tube catches the egg as it is expelled from the ovary and sweeps it toward the uterus. For pregnancy to occur, one sperm capable of fertilizing an egg must be present in the tube at the time of ovulation. Fertilization takes place in the Fallopian tube.

In the week following fertilization, the fertilized egg slowly moves toward the uterus, where it implants on the uterine wall. The internal surface of the Fallopian tube is lined with very delicate cells that contain fine, hairlike structures called *cilia*. Cilia sweep the egg and developing embryo down the tube, into the uterus.

72. *How do the cilia affect fertility?*

Even though the tubes can look normal on a hysterogram or laparoscopy, they may be damaged from a previous infection or from endometriosis.

Damage may be so minimal that it is not apparent in tests normally done for infertility. Yet the damage is enough to prevent conception.

It's impossible at this time to examine cilia without actually removing the tube. Minor damage may not be apparent, which may account for a woman's "unexplained" infertility.

73. *What are the major causes of tubal damage?*

One major cause of tubal damage is an infection called *salpingitis* that results in an inflammation or infection of the Fallopian tube. Salpingitis may be part of the more generalized infection involving tubes, uterus and ovaries called *PID*. See page 138.

74. *What is the most common cause of PID?*

Years ago, the most common cause was gonorrhea. Today, researchers believe chlamydial infections are the most common cause of PID. Chlamydial infections are more common than syphilis, gonorrhea and herpes *combined!* Other bacteria commonly found in the body, such as staphylococcus and streptococcus, can also cause PID.

75. *What are the symptoms of PID?*

The most common symptoms are low abdominal pain and fever. If the infection is more severe, nausea and vomiting may occur. There may also be a discharge from the cervix.

76. *When do symptoms occur?*

Symptoms may occur at any time but often first appear at the end of your period. Bacteria use the menstrual blood as a source of nourishment to multiply and grow. Menstrual blood is similar to material used in the laboratory when bacteria is grown on culture plates.

77. *How and when is PID treated?*

The sooner PID is treated with antibiotics, the less likely it is to cause permanent damage. If the infection is serious, it may require several days of hospitalization because antibiotics are given intravenously.

78. *How do these bacteria get into the Fallopian tube?*

Bacteria can get into the Fallopian tube in either of two ways. It can enter the tube from the blood supply to the tubes or it can enter in an ascending infection, which starts in the cervix and progresses to the uterus, then the Fallopian tubes. The cervical infection is often contracted from sexual contact with someone who carries the bacteria that causes PID.

Today, a common problem is PID associated with an IUD. With an IUD, bacteria can be transmitted from the vagina and cervix into the uterus by the IUD string.

79. *What are other causes of PID?*

Tuberculosis frequently caused permanent tubal damage in the past.

80. *Can other bacteria damage the Fallopian tube?*

Bacteria, such as mycoplasma, may also cause severe damage to Fallopian tubes.

81. *How else can a tube be damaged?*

Fallopian tubes can be damaged from any type of abdominal infection or from surgery. For instance, a ruptured appendix, in which the infection from the appendix reaches the outside of the tubes and ovaries, might cause scar tissue and adhesions on the Fallopian tubes.

82. *What problems can an IUD cause?*

Women who use IUDs for birth control are 4 to 9 times more likely to develop PID compared to women in the general population. Often an IUD doesn't cause an infection, but when a woman gets an infection with an IUD in place, the infection appears to be more severe.

83. *How common are IUD infections?*

Most women with IUDs do not get infections, especially if they have only one sexual partner.

84. *What if a woman has more than one sexual partner?*

With several sexual partners, a woman exposes herself to many different types of bacteria that may increase the chance of getting an infection. The multiple-partner factor applies to tubal infections in general but appears to be a major factor in women with IUDs.

85. *How does an infection damage the tubes?*

Bacteria causes an inflammation in the tubes that can affect the tubes in many ways. Inflammation can

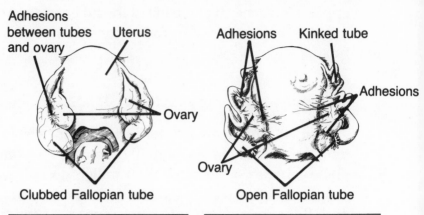

Adhesions
between tubes Uterus
and ovary

Adhesions   Kinked tube

Adhesions

Ovary

Ovary

Clubbed Fallopian tube

Open Fallopian tube

Uterus with blocked Fallo-
pian tubes and adhesions be-
tween tubes and ovaries.

Uterus with kinked Fallo-
pian tubes (from adhesions)
and adhesions between tubes
and ovaries. Fallopian tubes
are open.

cause damage to cilia, preventing the egg from being swept down the Fallopian tube. It can also block the end of the tube with scar tissue that forms as the body fights off infection. This is called *clubbing of the tubes;* it destroys the fimbria, which picks up the egg as it comes from the ovary. See illustrations above.

86. *Can a mild infection cause infertility?*

Yes, a mild infection may cause adhesions. Recent reports indicate a "silent" infection (one without symptoms) may cause as much damage as severe PID.

87. *What is an adhesion?*

An adhesion is a band of scar tissue that connects two pieces of tissue.

88. *What kind of problems do adhesions cause?*

Adhesions can attach the tube to the uterus, to another part of the tube (causing a kink in the tube) or to the ovary. This may prevent the tube from moving properly to get into position to catch the egg or stop the fertilized egg from entering the uterus, resulting in an ectopic pregnancy.

89. *What about severe PID?*

Severe pelvic infections can be a serious problem. They can be life threatening and may require a hysterectomy and salpingoophorectomy.

90. *Will medication heal adhesions and scar tissue?*

No. The only way to free adhesions and scar tissue is by surgery. If your doctor suspects damage to your tubes, he may suggest laparoscopy to look directly at them to see if there are blockage or adhesions.

91. *What can be done about minor adhesions?*

If adhesions are minor, they can be severed through the laparoscope. Recently, a laser beam has been used through a laparoscope to sever adhesions.

92. *What if adhesions are severe?*

If adhesions are severe, major surgery through an abdominal incision is necessary to attempt to open the tubes and free adhesions.

93. *What is this surgery called?*

The surgery is called a *tuboplasty*. It requires 3 to 5 days in the hospital and another 2 to 6 weeks recovery at home.

94. *What is the success rate of tuboplasty?*

It depends on the severity of the adhesions and blockage. Women who have only a few adhesions that cause a small bend in the tube have an excellent chance of becoming pregnant. If adhesions are severe and tubes are blocked, the success rate is not good.

95. *What complications can result from this surgery?*

Complications include infections, blood loss, risk of anesthesia, and adhesions and scar tissue forming from the surgical procedure.

OVARIAN FACTORS

96. *How is ovulation involved in fertility?*

Ovulation is the process by which the egg is expelled from the ovary. After ovulation occurs, the fimbria sweep the egg into the tube. Fertilization occurs in the Fallopian tube, where the sperm and egg meet. After fertilization, the egg is swept down the tube and into the uterus where it embeds itself. If there are any problems with this ovulation process, you may not be able to achieve pregnancy.

97. *What abnormalities can prevent ovulation?*

Ovulation is the end result of the interaction between hormones from the hypothalmus, the pituitary gland and the ovaries. Dysfunction of any of these glands can result in failure of the ovary to expel the egg. Other hormone-producing glands, such as the adrenal gland and thyroid gland, can also affect this process. Abnormalities of these glands must be considered when ovulation does not occur.

98. *What is a hormone imbalance?*

If you have a hormone imbalance, it means hormones work improperly or are produced inappropriately. This is the reason various blood tests, such as testosterone, DHEAS, cortisol, FSH, LH, thyroid profile and prolactin, may be ordered during your fertility investigation.

99. *How will I know if I am ovulating?*

If you have regular menstrual cycles at 26 to 32 days, you are probably ovulating on a regular basis. Occasionally pain at ovulation time (mittleschmerz) may occur. Other signs of an ovulatory cycle are premenstrual bloating, fluid retention and moodiness. Your doctor may become suspicious that you are not ovulating if you occasionally miss a period or say, "I'm regular, but I only have a period every other month."

100. *What can be done during an infertility investigation to determine ovulation?*

Several things may be done. Taking and recording your basal body temperature is the most common way to determine if ovulation occurs. Other methods to determine ovulation include performing an endometrial biopsy or checking a serum-progesterone level after suspected ovulation.

101. *Are there any other methods to determine ovulation?*

There are several new tests available. OvuStick, First Response and OvuTime are urine tests to do at home. They predict the sudden rise of LH, which precedes ovulation by 12 to 36 hours.

These tests are expensive for routine use and may not be totally reliable. They are usually recommended for predicting ovulation ahead of time when timed intercourse is difficult or when artificial insemination is necessary. The use of ultrasound can also be useful in predicting ovulation in some women.

102. *What is the Stein-Leventhal Syndrome?*

This syndrome is a hormone disorder that can cause irregular ovulation. It often occurs in women who are obese and who have excessive body hair. These two characteristics are associated with irregular ovulation and menstruation. Ovaries often have a thick capsule around them filled with small follicular (preovulation) cysts. Infertility blood studies show a slightly higher-than-normal serum testosterone along with an elevated serum LH.

103. *What can be done if ovulation is not occurring?*

A fertility drug, clomiphene citrate, can be given to make you ovulate. You may know this medication by its trade names Clomid and Serophene.

104. *How does it work?*

Clomiphene citrate is a synthetic hormone that stimulates the hypothalamus and pituitary glands to secrete higher levels of FSH and LH. FSH stimulates the egg to develop in the ovary, and LH causes the egg to be expelled from the ovary.

105. *How is this medication taken?*

It is usually started on the fifth day of the menstrual cycle; it is taken for 5 days. The first day of menstrual flow is considered day 1 of the cycle, so you take one pill a day on days 5 through 9. Most women respond to one pill a day for 5 days if they have irregular cycles. In some cases, a dose of two pills a day is needed for 5 days.

106. *How high a dose can I take?*

This depends on what your doctor recommends. The maximum recommended dose is 5 pills a day (250mg) for 5 days, but this dose may be increased under certain conditions.

107. *What if clomiphene citrate does not work?*

Clomiphene citrate may be combined with HCG

(human chorionic gonadotropin), which is very similar to LH. The HCG is given by injection about day 15 or 16 of the cycle. This combination of drugs may trigger ovulation shortly after it is given.

108. *What are the possible side effects of clomiphene citrate?*

It may cause breast tenderness, hair loss, hot flashes, bloating, mild depression or a sensation of seeing halos around lights. The most serious side effect is overstimulation of the ovaries, resulting in large ovarian cysts.

109. *How can these side effects be avoided?*

In most cases, they may be avoided by starting at the lowest possible dose of clomiphene and gradually working up to higher doses if lower doses do not work. Rarely a large cyst can form with the smallest recommended dosage.

110. *Are side effects permanent?*

No permanent side effects have been reported. Symptoms disappear after the medicine is discontinued.

111. *Can clomiphene citrate cause multiple pregnancies?*

Clomiphene citrate is *not* the drug you read about when people have five or six babies. That drug is Pergonal. Clomiphene citrate has a 6 to 8% chance of twins—6 out of 100 women will have twins. Triplets are possible but rare. Twins born to women taking clomiphene citrate are fraternal; they come from two different eggs.

112. *Does clomiphene citrate cause birth defects?*

The frequency of birth defects is not any higher if you take clomiphene citrate than if you conceive on your own.

113. *What if clomiphene citrate, or combining it with HCG, doesn't work?*

If this treatment doesn't work, you are usually given Pergonal.

114. *What is Pergonal?*

Pergonal is a preparation of FSH, and it is the most powerful agent we have to induce ovulation. It is very potent and potentially dangerous if not used properly. This drug may cause five, six or even seven fetuses to develop.

115. *How is Pergonal given?*

Pergonal is given by injection starting at the end of menstruation. You are checked daily with a pelvic exam, ultrasound and blood tests to make sure your ovaries are not being overstimulated.

When your estrogen reaches a certain level, HCG is given to trigger ovulation. You are asked to have intercourse on the day HCG is given to make sure sperm are present in the tube at the time of ovulation.

The trick in using Pergonal is to give HCG at the *right time*—when the estrogen level is in the range indicating only one ripe egg is present. An ultrasound exam before giving HCG has helped avoid multiple births and improved results.

116. *How expensive is Pergonal?*

It can be very expensive! Daily doctor visits, ultrasound exams and serum-estrogen blood tests can be $1,000 or more to trigger ovulation for *one month.*

117. *Does ovulation guarantee pregnancy?*

Even when ovulation occurs using Pergonal, there is no guarantee of pregnancy. All other factors involved in infertility should be ruled out as a cause before Pergonal is used.

118. *Do all doctors administer Pergonal?*

No; not all doctors are qualified to give Pergonal. A doctor must have experience in using this drug because of potential complications. He should be able to evaluate serum-estrogen levels in a few hours and have an ultrasound machine. Pergonal is usually administered by large infertility clinics.

119. *What are the potential complications of Pergonal?*

The biggest complication is overstimulation of the ovaries. This can result in formation of ovarian cysts the size of a basketball—surgery may be needed if the cysts do not resolve on their own.

120. *Are there any dangers if I become pregnant with Pergonal?*

If you ovulate and become pregnant, there is the danger of multiple pregnancies and the danger of premature birth and its complications. Often babies are born so prematurely they weigh only 1 to 2 pounds and have little chance of survival.

121. *What is GNRH, and how is it used in infertility?*

GNRH is gonadotropin-releasing hormone. It is produced by the hypothalmus, which stimulates the pituitary gland to produce FSH and LH.

Synthetic GNRH can be given to women with certain types of ovulation disorders, such as those who do not respond to clomiphene citrate. It is used in some cases where Pergonal was previously used and failed, with good results. Some doctors are trying GNRH before using Pergonal.

122. *How is GNRH given?*

GNRH is given by injection—intramuscularly or intravenously. A fertility pump has been used with success by some researchers. A fertility pump is the common name for a device developed for use as an insulin pump. This small pump is inserted under the skin where it releases a substance continuously into the bloodstream. The pump's use in infertility has been with GNRH; it is still considered experimental.

123. *What are other causes of ovulation disorders?*

In recent years, prolactin has been found to play a large part in ovulation disorders. Hyperprolactinemia (elevated serum prolactin) is believed to be the underlying cause of infertility in as many as 33% of all women who seek treatment for infertility. Almost all women with an increased prolactin level are infertile.

124. *What is prolactin?*

Prolactin is a hormone secreted by the pituitary gland. It enables you to secrete milk and nurse after you have a baby.

Unlike FSH and LH, which are controlled by stimulating factors from the hypothalmus, prolactin is controlled by certain prolactin-inhibiting factors from the hypothalmus. Estrogen and thyroid hormone may also have an influence on stimulating prolactin secretion from the pituitary gland.

If the pathway between the hypothalmus and pituitary gland are cut off, it causes a decrease in FSH and LH and an increase in prolactin because of the removal of the. prolactin-inhibiting factor. With a decrease in FSH and LH and an increase in prolactin, the result is amenorrhea-galactorrhea.

125. *What are the symptoms of high levels of prolactin?*

The most common symptom is leakage of fluid from your breasts, which is called *galactorrhea*. Irregular periods and amenorrhea are other common symptoms. The condition of amenorrhea with galactorrhea should alert your doctor that an elevated prolactin level is probably present.

126. *How does prolactin interfere with ovulation?*

Prolactin prevents the appropriate amounts of FSH and LH from being released by the pituitary gland.

127. *What causes a high prolactin level?*

The most frequent cause of an elevated prolactin level is a small pituitary gland tumor called a *pituitary adenoma* or *microadenoma*.

128. *Are there other causes of high levels of prolactin?*

Yes. Sharply elevated prolactin levels are normally found during the latter stages of pregnancy and post-partum. Serum prolactin remains elevated if you breast-feed. Increased prolactin can also occur naturally during sleep, intercourse and nipple stimulation. Drugs, such as potent tranquilizers, anti-depressants, estrogen, blood-pressure medication and birth-control pills, can cause increased prolactin levels. Hypothyroidism may also cause galactorrhea.

129. *How are pituitary adenomas diagnosed?*

In addition to the physical symptoms of irregular periods, amenorrhea, galactorrhea and headaches, double vision and visual-field defects may be present from pressure from the tumor on the optic nerves.

An elevated prolactin level is also present. A CT scan or special X-rays of the pituitary gland will show if a pituitary-gland tumor is present.

130. *How are pituitary adenomas treated?*

A new drug, bromocryptine (Parlodel), can be given to suppress the prolactin level and shrink a tumor. Recent reports have shown bromocryptine is useful in treating small and large tumors of the pituitary gland. If the tumor does not respond to bromocryptine, it should be removed surgically.

131. *Will ovulation return to normal?*

Ovulation usually returns to normal after Parlodel is given or the pituitary tumor is removed.

132. *Are there other uses for Parlodel in infertility?*

Recent studies and clinical experience have demonstrated that even though a random prolactin level will be normal, there can be a transient, sporadic elevation of prolactin that has been associated with infertility. Bromocryptine has been tried and has resulted in some success in "unexplained" infertility or in women with "high-normal" levels of prolactin.

133. *Can anything be done surgically to help ovulation?*

Before clomiphene citrate came into use, ovarian wedge resection was often performed.

134. *What is an ovarian wedge resection?*

It is a major surgical procedure in which a wedge is removed from the ovary; about 20 to 35% of each ovary is removed.

135. *What does an ovarian wedge resection do?*

It decreases estrogen production of the ovaries and stimulates production of FSH and LH, allowing the ovary to function normally.

136. *Why isn't ovarian wedge resection done as often today?*

Clomiphene citrate accomplishes the same thing without surgery and with better results. Ovarian wedge resection is occasionally done when you fail to respond to clomiphene citrate. It is used most commonly in cases of Stein-Leventhal Syndrome that are unresponsive to clomiphene citrate.

137. *Can the ovaries stop functioning earlier than expected?*

Yes. There is a condition called *premature menopause* or *premature ovarian failure* that results in typical menopausal symptoms at an early age. Symptoms may occur as early as age 25 to 35.

138. *What are the symptoms of premature ovarian failure?*

Symptoms of this condition are similar to those of menopause. They include hot flashes and flushes, amenorrhea, vaginal dryness and breast atrophy.

139. *How is premature ovarian failure diagnosed?*

A serum-FSH test is markedly elevated. There is no feedback of estrogen to the pituitary gland, so the FSH level rises.

140. *Is there any treatment for this condition?*

No, there isn't. Rarely, the condition can persist for a few months or a year, then spontaneously resolve itself for no known reason. Estrogen replacement can be prescribed for the hot flashes and vaginal atrophy, but it will not restore fertility.

141. *Are there any genetic disorders that prevent ovulation?*

Yes. Several abnormalities occur in which a woman cannot produce eggs. These conditions are rare; we mention only the most common of these—*Turner's Syndrome.*

142. *What is Turner's Syndrome?*

This condition is caused by the presence of only one X chromosome in a woman. A woman with Turner's Syndrome is called an XO female. Normally, a woman has two X chromosomes (XX), and a man has one X chromosome and one Y chromosome (XY). A woman with Turner's Syndrome has no ovaries, so she doesn't produce estrogen or ovulate. Another name for Turner's Syndrome is *gonadal dysgenesis.*

143. *How common is Turner's Syndrome?*

It occurs in 0.04% (4 in 10,000) of all newborn females.

144. *How is Turner's Syndrome discovered?*

It may be discovered at birth, when a newborn female may show typical characteristics of the syndrome, including loose skin folds at the nape of the neck, edema of the back of the hands and feet, coarctation of the aorta and a horseshoe-shaped kidney. If it is not discovered in a newborn, Turner's Syndrome often goes undetected until puberty, when amenorrhea and lack of sexual development become obvious.

A woman with Turner's Syndrome is unusually short (48 to 58 inches tall) and has no breast or sexual development. She exhibits loose skin folds at the back of the neck and a broad, shieldlike chest with widely spaced nipples. In addition, she may have a wide carrying angle at her elbows and possibly heart and kidney abnormalities.

145. *How is Turner's Syndrome diagnosed?*

In addition to physical characteristics, it can be diagnosed with elevated serum FSH and the discovery of streaked ovaries during a laparoscopy exam. A chromosomal analysis is then ordered, and the suspected XO female is usually confirmed.

146. *Is a woman with Turner's Syndrome sterile?*

Yes. She has only small bands of scar tissue called *streaks* where ovaries are normally located. There are no eggs present in the streaks, and she does not produce estrogen and will not develop sexually without taking estrogen. Breasts develop and periods start if she takes estrogen and progesterone, but she will still remain sterile.

147. *Can Turner's Syndrome be treated?*

Other than replacing estrogen and progesterone, there is no treatment. Nothing can be done to make a woman with Turner's Syndrome fertile.

7

What Is Endometriosis?

Endometriosis is a common disorder found in about 20% of all women who are infertile. It appears to be on the increase. Today, many women delay having children until a later age, and this may contribute to the increased rate of endometriosis. Endometriosis is less common in societies in which girls marry young and have children at an earlier age.

1. *What is endometriosis?*

Endometriosis is a disease in which the tissue that normally lines the endometrium becomes implanted and starts to grow in other places in the body.

2. *Where does this tissue become implanted?*

It usually is found on the ovaries and ligaments that support the uterus (uterosacral and broad ligaments).

Endometriosis is also found on the Fallopian tubes, bladder, small intestine, rectum, cervix and vagina. Rarely, endometrial growths are found on distant organs, such as the lung.

3. *How does endometrial tissue become implanted where it doesn't belong?*

We don't know for sure, but there are several theories. One is that the glands have been there since birth; for some reason under the influence of estrogen, they start to grow. Another is when a woman has her period, the uterine lining sheds "backward" through the Fallopian tubes and goes into the pelvic cavity where it implants on the ovaries and ligaments and starts to grow as if it was inside the uterus. A third theory is that tissue gets into the bloodstream from the uterine vessels and ends up in a distant organ, such as the lung. See illustration on opposite page.

4. *How does endometriosis interfere with conception?*

It can interfere in many ways. If endometriosis is severe enough, it can cause adhesions that block or severely limit the movement of Fallopian tubes. Endometriosis may get into the ovaries and interfere with normal hormone production and ovulation. It can cause interference with movement of the cilia and prevent a fertilized egg from being swept down into the uterus. This may result in the egg becoming blocked half way down the Fallopian tube, which results in a tubal pregnancy.

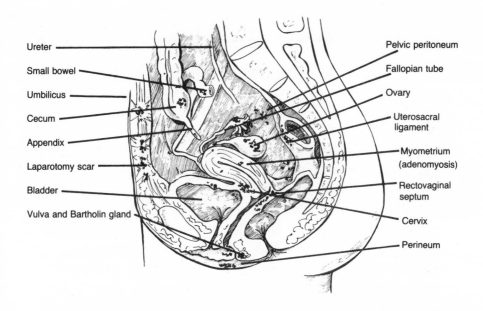

Various sites of endometriosis.

5. *If I have endometriosis, does it mean I won't be able to become pregnant?*

Definitely not; many women with endometriosis do become pregnant. Although 70% of all women with endometriosis have a fertility problem, about 60% of them can become pregnant with appropriate treatment. Out of 10 women with endometriosis, 3 will become pregnant without treatment. With treatment, an additional 4 will become pregnant.

6. *What are symptoms of endometriosis?*

Endometriosis is a very unpredictable disease. Some women with extensive endometriosis have very few symptoms; other women with minimal endometriosis have severe symptoms. The most common symptom is severe menstrual cramps. In severe cases, pain lasts longer than during a period; sometimes it lasts all month long.

If the ovaries become involved, they can become as large as a grapefruit. This can cause pressure in the pelvis and irregular periods. Other symptoms include painful bowel movements and painful urination if the colon and bladder become involved. Painful intercourse (dyspareunia) can also be a symptom.

7. *What causes these symptoms?*

When you have your period each month, tissue that normally lines the uterus is shed with your period. When you have endometriosis, the tissue present elsewhere in the pelvis, such as on the ovary or ligaments, has nowhere to go. So each month, when you have your period, tissue swells and bleeds, which causes pain.

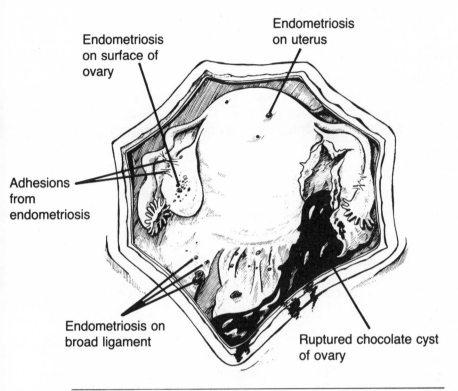

Endometriosis
on surface of
ovary

Endometriosis
on uterus

Adhesions
from
endometriosis

Endometriosis on
broad ligament

Ruptured chocolate cyst
of ovary

Uterus with endometriosis and chocolate cyst (endometrioma) that has ruptured.

8. *What happens when tissue swells and bleeds?*

Because there is no where for the blood to go, it begins to accumulate in little cysts.

9. *Do these cysts cause problems?*

Cysts can grow large and become filled with old,

dried blood—they are called *chocolate cysts*. Chocolate refers to the dried blood that accumulates in the cysts. See illustration on previous page.

10. *Is endometriosis hereditary?*

There is a tendency for endometriosis to run in families. If your mother or sister has endometriosis, your chances are 7 times greater that you will also develop it. Endometriosis is normally found in 1% of all women; it occurs in 7% of women who have a mother or sister with endometriosis.

11. *Is endometriosis prevalent at a certain age?*

It generally occurs in women over 30 years old who have postponed childbirth, but it can also occur at an earlier age. Endometriosis is often called the *career woman's disease*. Career women concentrate their efforts during their 20s pursuing education and careers rather than having children. If you delay having children, you increase your chances of having endometriosis.

12. *How is endometriosis diagnosed?*

Your doctor may suspect it if you have a history of painful periods or painful intercourse. He may also suspect it if he finds tenderness or irregularities of the ovaries or ligaments during a pelvic examination.

The best way to diagnose endometriosis is by laparoscopy. Your doctor can look directly into the pelvis to see if endometriosis is present. The condition may be discovered when a laparoscopy exam is performed as part of an infertility investigation.

13. *What is the best treatment for endometriosis?*

Treatment is usually one of two choices—surgical or medical. It usually depends on whether the endometriosis is mild or severe.

14. *What is the treatment for mild endometriosis?*

If it is very mild, no treatment may be necessary. If only a few glands or cysts are seen at a laparoscopy exam, the endometriosis can be cauterized with a special instrument. Laser beams have also been used during laparoscopy to treat endometriosis.

15. *What if the endometriosis is severe?*

If large ovarian cysts, extensive scar tissue and adhesions have formed, surgery may be needed. This is major surgery, with a full abdominal incision; it removes the cysts, frees the adhesions and cauterizes remaining endometriosis implants. It is called *conservative surgery* because fertility is preserved.

16. *Is hospitalization required for endometriosis surgery?*

When major surgery is required, 3 to 5 days in the hospital is necessary. You will need to recover at home for another 2 to 6 weeks. If only laparoscopy is performed, it usually can be done on a 1-day hospital stay.

17. *Is it common to have surgery more than once for endometriosis?*

Several surgeries may be necessary because endometriosis can recur. It may also be advisable to have a laparoscopy exam several months after surgery if you haven't become pregnant. The purpose of a repeat laparoscopy is to see if there is any residual endometriosis and to cut any adhesions that may have formed from the previous surgery.

18. *What is the medical treatment of endometriosis?*

The goal is to prevent you from having periods so tissue that is present does not bleed. The most popular drug for this is the birth-control pill, which allows tissue to dissolve and disappear.

19. *How is the pill taken for treatment of endometriosis?*

Instead of taking the pill cyclically (3 weeks on, 1 week off), the pill is taken continuously without a break for 6 to 9 months.

20. *What if bleeding occurs?*

If a woman has breakthrough bleeding, two pills a day are taken and possibly more.

21. *Are there side effects from taking birth-control pills continuously?*

There can be side effects from taking them continuously. Side effects include nausea, fluid retention, bloating, weight gain and breakthrough bleeding. Anyone who should not take the pill for birth control should not take it for endometriosis. If you have a history of heart disease, blood clots or high blood pressure, do not take birth-control pills. Taking birth-control pills for endometriosis is often called *creating a pseudopregnancy* (false pregnancy).

22. *What is pseudopregnancy?*

Pseudopregnancy causes symptoms similar to pregnancy—no periods, feeling nauseated, bloating, weight gain and other pregnancy symptoms. The purpose of creating a pseudopregnancy is to have you go at least 9 months without a period.

23. *What other medications can be taken?*

Medications that contain only progesterone (birth-control pills contain estrogen and progesterone), such as Depo-provera, can also be used. Depo-provera can be given by injection every month.

24. *Are there side effects from Depo-provera?*

The disadvantage of Depo-provera is that your hormones may become oversuppressed, and you may not ovulate for 1 to 2 *years* after stopping the medication.

25. *What is the most common medication used for endometriosis today?*

Presently, danazol is the most common drug used; it

is often sold under the brand name Danocrine. Instead of creating a pseudopregnancy, danazol creates a pseudomenopause.

26. *What is pseudomenopause?*

Pseudomenopause is the condition in which you do not have periods because the amounts of FSH, LH and estrogen are reduced. The condition is similar to what happens when a woman goes through menopause.

27. *How does danazol work?*

It interferes with the release of FSH and LH from the pituitary gland. This prevents the ovaries from producing estrogen needed to stimulate endometriosis.

28. *What are the side effects of danazol?*

Danazol is related to male hormones, so most of the side effects are similar to taking testosterone. Side effects include weight gain, an increased appetite, acne, oily skin, male-type hair growth, deepening of the voice and a decrease in breast size. Usually these side effects are not as severe as they sound.

29. *Are side effects temporary?*

Yes, but it may take several months after you stop the medication before they disappear.

30. *How long do I have to take medication?*

Once you agree to medical treatment, whether it is birth-control pills or danazol, it's best to continue for 6 to 9 months.

31. *Can I become pregnant during this time?*

Ideally, you won't have a period or vaginal bleeding while you are on the medication, so you won't be able to become pregnant.

32. *If I have endometriosis, what are my chances of becoming pregnant with or without treatment?*

It depends on how severe the endometriosis is. Thirty to 40% of all women with mild endometriosis eventually become pregnant without treatment. Pregnancy rates following use of danazol or birth-control pills or after conservative surgery are in the 40-to-60% range. Often, surgical and medical treatment are used together, with even greater success. About 70% of all infertile women with endometriosis who seek treatment become pregnant.

33. *I've heard that pregnancy can cure endometriosis. Is this true?*

Yes. The high progesterone levels produced by the placenta during pregnancy help dissolve endometriosis. You don't have periods during the 9 months you're pregnant; this is also achieved with medical treatment, so pregnancy is an excellent cure for endometriosis.

34. *If pregnancy is the cure, can I get pregnant again if I have endometriosis?*

Most women find it easier to become pregnant after having a baby. However, occasionally a woman develops endometriosis *after* having several children.

35. *Will treatment for endometriosis cure pain as well as improve my chances to become pregnant?*

Hopefully, taking birth-control pills or danazol relieves the pain associated with endometriosis and improves your chances to become pregnant when medication is discontinued. Surgical treatment should also alleviate pain if the endometriosis is removed and the area cauterized.

36. *Is there a permanent treatment for endometriosis?*

Endometriosis is dependent on the estrogen production from the ovaries, so a total hysterectomy with removal of the uterus, tubes and ovaries may be needed if all else fails. This results in sterility. If a woman is still having symptoms from endometriosis after she stops having children, she should consider having a hysterectomy.

8

How Is Infertility in a Man Diagnosed?

When it is suspected that your husband may have a fertility problem, you will probably discover it from tests your physician orders. You may have questions about the tests and what their results mean.

This section is devoted to how infertility in men is diagnosed. The causes and treatments of male infertility are covered in the next section, which begins on page 192.

1. *How is male infertility diagnosed?*

Infertility in a man is diagnosed by obtaining semen for analysis. A semen analysis is a laboratory test that measures the sperm count and other important qualities of semen and sperm. If the test is normal, further testing of the man is unnecessary. If it is abnormal, additional studies are necessary.

2. *What is the difference between sperm and semen?*

Sperm means sperm cells; *semen* means the total content of the ejaculate—the fluid and sperm. An individual sperm cell fertilizes the egg.

3. *Where do sperm and semen come from?*

Sperm come from the testicles. Semen is produced by the seminal vesicles, prostate gland and Cowper's glands.

4. *What is a normal sperm count?*

In the past, about 60 million sperm/cc (5cc is equivalent to 1 teaspoon) was considered normal. If other factors, such as motility, viability and morphology of the sperm, are normal studies show a man's fertility doesn't increase unless his sperm count falls below 20 million sperm in 1 cc. It is considered normal if 40 to 60 million sperm are present in the *total* ejaculate.

5. *What are the qualities of the semen and sperm that are important?*

Qualities of the semen include its volume, thickness, alkalinity, signs of infection and the presence of fructose. Qualities of the sperm include motility, morphology, viability, clumping and agglutination.

6. *What if no sperm are present?*

Complete absence of sperm in a semen analysis may

be from failure of the testicles to produce sperm or from a blockage in the ductal system (epididymis and vas deferens), preventing their escape.

7. *Why is the presence of fructose important?*

Fructose is a type of sugar normally produced in the epididymis, which is part of the ductal system in a man. If fructose is present in a semen analysis, it means the ductal system is open. If fructose is not present, it means it is blocked.

8. *What is normal motility?*

Motility refers to the ability of sperm to move spontaneously. Movement should be in a forward direction, especially when observed in cervical mucus. In a semen analysis, at least 60% of sperm should still be active and moving 1 hour after obtaining the specimen.

9. *What is normal viability?*

Viability of sperm refers to the number of live sperm present in the semen specimen. It's normal to have a certain percentage of dead sperm, but at least 60% of them should be alive.

10. *What is morphology?*

Morphology refers to how the sperm look. Every man has a certain percentage of abnormal-looking sperm. In a normal analysis, at least 65% of the sperm are normal.

11. *What does clumping of sperm indicate?*

If sperm clump together, it can be a sign of an infection in the prostate gland.

12. *What is agglutination of sperm?*

Agglutination is a situation in which the heads or tails of sperm adhere to each other. This occurs when a man is allergic to his own sperm. See illustrations on opposite page.

13. *What is the normal volume of the ejaculate?*

A normal volume is between 2cc and 5cc.

14. *What is liquefaction and viscosity of semen?*

Semen is ejaculated in a liquid state. It immediately becomes very thick and gummy, then liquefies within 20 minutes. The process when semen changes from the thick, gummy state to the liquid state is called *liquefaction;* it enables sperm to enter the cervical mucus. The thickness of the semen after it liquefies is called *viscosity.* Occasionally, the semen does not liquefy and remains very thick; this decreases the motility of the sperm.

15. *What factors in a semen analysis are most important?*

Sperm motility and morphology appear to have the best correlation with fertility. The actual number of sperm—the sperm count—appears to be less important than researchers once believed.

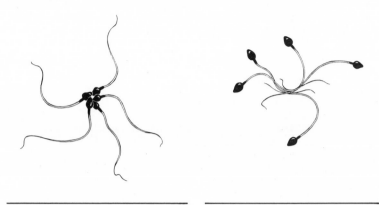

Head-to-head agglutination.   *Tail-to-tail agglutination.*

16. *Where is a semen analysis done?*

Your physician will order a semen analysis; if you are seeing a doctor for infertility, it is usually ordered by him. A semen analysis should be performed by a laboratory experienced in performing semen analyses, either in the doctor's office or in a medical laboratory where trained technicians are available.

17. *How is a semen specimen obtained?*

It is usually obtained by masturbation and is collected in a clean, dry container. A specimen can be collected at the laboratory or at home and brought to the laboratory within 30 to 60 minutes. It must be kept warm (not hot) by keeping it close to the body while taking it to the laboratory.

18. *Are there other things we should be aware of before the test?*

Do not have intercourse 2 to 3 days before collecting the specimen. Too-frequent ejaculations, especially in a man with a borderline sperm count, may reduce the sperm count.

19. *What about infrequent ejaculations?*

A man who has intercourse once or twice a month may have a specimen with many dead sperm with poor motility. If you're trying to become pregnant, have intercourse once or twice a week during the month and every other day at midcycle.

20. *What if religious or personal reasons prevent my husband from obtaining a semen specimen by masturbation?*

If it is not feasible to obtain the specimen by masturbation, a condom that does not contain substances to kill sperm may be used during intercourse. The specimen can be saved in the condom and brought to the laboratory.

21. *Will my husband have to repeat a semen analysis?*

Sometimes when the specimen reveals borderline results or the specimen does not correlate with the wife's post-coital test, a second or even third specimen may be required. Results of a semen analysis can change markedly in a short period of time. Your doctor will ask for a repeat semen analysis if it is necessary.

22. *Should my husband have any other tests?*

If the semen analysis is normal, no further testing is needed. If it's abnormal, other tests will be necessary.

23. *What type of doctor should my husband see for further infertility tests?*

Usually a urologist (a doctor who specializes in treating urinary tract problems in men and women) treats a man with infertility.

24. *What should my husband expect if he goes to a urologist for infertility?*

A complete medical and sexual history will be done. This includes a social history, such as occupation and activities, medications he may be taking and drug use. The doctor will also want to know if your husband ever had any urologic infections, genital injuries or past episodes of sexually transmitted diseases. A physical exam will be performed, with special attention to the scrotum, testicles, epididymis and vas deferens. If a prostate infection is suspected, a prostatic massage may be done to examine secretions from the prostate gland.

25. *What does the doctor look for when he examines him?*

He examines the testicles to see if they are of normal size and consistency or if unusual tenderness or swelling is present. He will exam your husband to see if he has a hydrocele or varicocele. See page 193.

26. *Are there any laboratory tests that will be performed?*

A urinalysis will be done to check for infection. A complete blood count and other pertinent kidney or liver tests may be ordered, depending on your husband's history and physical exam.

Screening hormone tests, such as dehydroepiandosterone sulfate (DHEAS), serum testosterone, prolactin, FSH and LH, may also be performed.

27. *What will abnormalities of these hormones indicate?*

They may indicate an abnormal secretion of hormones or possible tumors of the hypothalmus, pituitary, thyroid or adrenal glands. Hormone tests may reveal abnormal hormone production by the testicles.

28. *Are certain occupations associated with infertility?*

Yes. Men who work near blast furnaces in steel mills have been shown to have low sperm counts. Any occupation with prolonged exposure to heat will result in poor sperm production. Truck drivers who sit for long periods in tight jockey shorts often have decreased fertility.

29. *Can certain medications affect fertility?*

Any medication a man takes may affect his semen analysis. Common medications, such as antihistamines for allergies, antibiotics for urinary infections, medications for ulcers, tranquilizers and anti-depressants, may cause a decrease in the sperm count and sperm motility. In addition to the effect on sperm production, some medications may cause impotence, with a failure to sustain an erection or to ejaculate.

30. *Does marijuana affect fertility?*

In small, infrequent doses, marijuana probably does not affect sperm production. Heavy use of marijuana can suppress sperm production and decrease a man's sex drive. This can be an important factor in men who have a borderline semen analysis. Avoid using marijuana when trying to conceive.

31. *Does alcohol affect fertility?*

Alcohol probably does not affect sperm production if used in small amounts. Heavy use of alcohol decreases intercourse frequency and may cause impotence. Chronic use of alcohol may cause damage to the liver, which affects the way sex hormones are excreted from the body. This may result in poor sperm production.

32. *Does DES exposure in a man affect fertility?*

Yes, it can. Years ago, DES was given to pregnant

women who threatened to miscarry. It is now known many children born to these women later developed abnormalities of their reproductive systems. At first, the effect of DES was thought to be only on women, but today we know men also develop abnormalities. They may have abnormalities of their ductal systems (epididymis and vas deferens), with poor sperm development and decreased fertility.

33. *Can exposure to certain toxic chemicals affect fertility?*

Definitely. Sperm counts of men in the United States have fallen 20% since the last generation. This may be due to exposure to different toxins in the atmosphere and exposure to chemicals in the work-place. Hundreds of toxic chemicals are byproducts of industrial life and may affect sperm production.

34. *What occupations have the greatest risk?*

Medicine, dentistry, smelting, battery production, chemistry, agriculture, glass factories and aviation appear to have the highest risk. It's important for your doctor to know if there is a chance your husband has been exposed to toxic chemicals in his work environment.

35. *Can X-ray or other radiation exposure affect sperm production?*

X-ray exposure may have an effect. If a man works in an environment where X-rays are taken, he must wear protective shields during exposure. If someone needs radiation treatment, shielding the scrotal area is necessary if it doesn't interfere with treatment.

36. *What precautions can be taken to minimize the risk from exposure to toxic chemicals?*

If there is a question about the safety of the work environment, such as exposure to toxic chemicals, your state's Department of Health can give you information about the type of exposure and risks involved.

37. *Can occupational exposure to excess heat suppress sperm count?*

Yes; this has been well-established. Men who work in steel mills near hot blasting furnaces often have a low sperm count with poor motility and an increase in abnormally shaped sperm. Truck drivers who sit for long periods of time have also been shown to have similar semen qualities. This is believed to be a result of increased temperature in the scrotum. Any other type of work where there is exposure to excess heat may also suppress the sperm count.

38. *Can the type of underwear my husband wears affect fertility?*

Possibly. Tight, jockey-type shorts may cause a rise in the scrotal temperature, which affects the sperm count. The frequent wearing of athletic supporters may also affect sperm production.

39. *Can hot tubs, saunas and whirlpools affect fertility?*

In a man with a normal semen analysis, short exposure to heat under these conditions should have no affect on sperm production. In a man with a borderline semen analysis, exposure to excessive heat for long periods of time in a sauna or hot tub may affect sperm production.

A recent study has shown that sitting in a moderately heated hot tub (102F) resulted in a rapid drop in sperm count and penetration capability for the following 6 weeks. The effect appears to be more in the penetration capability of sperm, *not* in the count and motility. It took 7 weeks for everything to return to normal.

In view of this evidence, if you are experiencing infertility, it would be advisable for your husband to avoid hot tubs and saunas.

40. *What is agent orange?*

It is a powerful herbicide that was used in Vietnam to kill shrubbery in the jungle.

41. *Can past exposure to agent orange affect my husband's fertility?*

There have been reports of decreased sperm counts and an increase in stillbirths and birth defects in children fathered by men exposed to agent orange. Other studies have not confirmed this.

42. *What is a testicular biopsy?*

A small piece of tissue is removed from the testicle and examined under a microscope to help find the cause of a man's infertility. It is usually performed when the semen analysis reveals no sperm or very few sperm.

43. *Where is a testicular biopsy performed?*

It is usually performed in a doctor's office under local anesthesia or under general anesthesia as an outpatient in a hospital or surgical center.

44. *What does the doctor look for in a testicular biopsy?*

A testicular biopsy reveals if sperm-producing cells are present, if there is maturation arrest (cessation of sperm development) or if inflammation of the tubules of the testicles is present.

45. *What is maturation arrest?*

With maturation arrest, sperm do not progress past a very early stage of development—they do not mature. Sperm that are present are incapable of fertilizing an egg because of immaturity.

46. *Is there a treatment for maturation arrest?*

No, there is no treatment.

47. *What is the Sertoli-cell-only Syndrome?*

It is a condition in which there is a complete absence of sperm-producing cells. The Sertoli cell is a cell in the testicle that sperm depend on for nutrition. If it is the only cell seen on a biopsy, it means there are no sperm-producing cells—the man is sterile.

48. *Can the Sertoli-cell-only Syndrome be treated?*

No, there is no treatment.

49. *Can a man with maturation arrest or Sertoli-cell-only Syndrome have children?*

No; he is sterile. The only possible treatment would be for his wife to have donor insemination.

50. *What if a testicular biopsy is normal?*

If a testicular biopsy is normal and the semen analysis reveals no sperm, it indicates an obstruction of the ductal system (epididymis or vas deferens) after sperm leave the testicle.

51. *How can the doctor tell if there is an obstruction? What tests can he perform?*

A semen analysis will reveal an absence of fructose. In addition, the doctor can perform a procedure called *seminal vasography.*

52. *What is seminal vasography?*

It is a test in which a radiopaque dye (a dye that can be seen on X-ray) is injected into the vas deferens to see if the sperm ductal system is blocked. After the dye is injected into the vas deferens, an X-ray is taken so the ductal system can be seen.

53. *Is this test performed in the hospital?*

It is performed wherever the doctor has access to an X-ray machine—in his office or the X-ray department of a hospital.

9

What Are the Causes and Treatments of Infertility in a Man?

There are many causes of infertility in men—many causes are treatable, and many are not. Some causes can be treated with surgery, and others can be treated with hormones. Many methods of treatment that were commonly used in the past are no longer used because they have proved to be of little value. In this section, we will discuss the most common causes and treatments of male infertility.

1. *What is the most frequently diagnosed cause of male infertility?*

A varicocele is the most common, most treatable cause of male infertility. A varicocele accounts for about 50% of all known causes of male infertility.

2. *What are other causes of male infertility?*

About 25 to 30% of the causes include infections,

hormonal abnormalities, obstructive and non-obstructive azoospermia, and other reasons, such as medications. The remaining cases are termed "unknown" or "idiopathic" infertility. A large percentage of this idiopathic group may be attributable to the inability of sperm to penetrate the egg. Using the hamster-egg-penetration assay to diagnose this type of infertility may be helpful. See page 221.

3. *What is a varicocele?*

A varicocele is a group of varicose veins around the testicles in the scrotum. Ninety percent of all varicoceles are found in the left scrotum, but they may also be located on the right side or on both sides. See illustration on following page.

4. *How is a varicocele diagnosed?*

The first indication that a varicocele may be present is on a semen analysis. A large number of tapered and other abnormal-looking sperm, with a decrease in motility, is highly suggestive that a varicocele is present. The presence of a low sperm count, sperm with tapered heads and poor motility indicate a condition called a *stress pattern* on a semen analysis; it is commonly seen in men with a varicocele.

5. *How does a varicocele affect sperm production?*

There are several theories. The first is the increased blood in the dilated veins around the testicle raises the temperature of the testicles and decreases sperm qual-

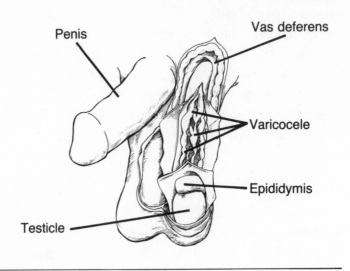

Male genitals with varicocele.

ity. A second theory is hormones from the adrenal gland, which connect with the varicocele, inhibit sperm production and maturation. Yet another theory is the increase in venous pressure from the dilated veins creates a shunting of blood into the arteries around the testicle, causing hypoxia (decreased oxygen supply) to the testicle.

6. *How common is a varicocele?*

Ten percent of *all* men have a varicocele. Not all men with varicoceles are infertile, but 40 to 50% of all men who go to a doctor for infertility have a varicocele.

7. *How is a varicocele treated?*

Surgery, called *spermatic vein ligation*, is the treatment. An incision is made in the lower abdomen to tie off the internal spermatic vein. Varicose veins around the testicles drain into the spermatic vein on their way back to the abdomen. After this vein is tied off, blood can no longer back up into the varicocele. *A varicocele is the most common, treatable cause of male infertility.*

Surgery takes about an hour, and the incision is similar to a hernia repair. It can be done on a 1-day stay in the hospital, but spending 1 or 2 nights in the hospital may be necessary if excessive pain or swelling are present. The use of the operating microscope and microsurgery has made varicocele surgery an even greater success.

8. *How successful is the surgery?*

Seventy to 80% of all men who have varicocele surgery have an improved semen analysis. Fifty to 60% of the men who have the operation eventually father children.

9. *How long does it take to find out if a spermatic vein ligation worked?*

It takes a minimum of 3 months before there is any change in the semen analysis. It takes 72 days from the time the sperm are first produced in the testicle until they mature and are expelled in the ejaculate. There may be gradual improvement in semen and sperm quality for up to 12 months following surgery.

10. *What is a hydrocele?*

It is a collection of fluid around the testicle. It usually

does not interfere with fertility unless it is very large and occurs on both sides.

11. *How is a hydrocele treated?*

Surgical removal of the hydrocele sac is necessary if it affects fertility.

12. *Can mumps affect a man's fertility?*

Mumps as a child does not affect fertility. About 1 in 4 adult men who gets mumps contracts *mumps orchitis* (inflammation of the testicles) and becomes permanently sterile.

13. *What are the symptoms of mumps orchitis?*

Symptoms include the usual symptom of mumps— swelling of the parotid gland (just below the ear). If testicles become infected when a man has mumps, they become very swollen, tender and painful. Mumps may involve one or both testicles. If only one is involved, the other testicle will be normal, with normal sperm production.

14. *Is there treatment for sterility from mumps orchitis?*

Unfortunately not. A small percentage of men will have a gradual return in their sperm production if the testicles were not markedly swollen. If a man is told he is sterile from a recent mumps orchitis, his semen analysis should be repeated later to see if there has been any recovery. Only 25% of men who get mumps get orchitis. Of those with orchitis, a small percentage may recover, even if both testicles are involved.

15. *Can injuries to the testicles cause infertility?*

Any severe injury to the scrotum or testicles that results in swelling or hematoma formation may result in permanent damage to sperm-producing cells of the testicle. For sterility to occur, damage would have to be in both testicles. There is no treatment for this type of sterility.

16. *How often are low sperm counts caused by trauma?*

The usual bumps and bruises a man gets participating in sports do not cause damage to the testicles. An injury must be severe enough to cause marked swelling; even then permanent damage is rare.

17. *Can an injury from a previous operation affect fertility?*

If a man had a hernia repair as an infant or young adult, the blood supply to the testicles could have been compromised. This could cause testicular atrophy as an adult.

18. *What is testicular atrophy?*

With testicular atrophy, the testicle "dies" and shrivels up from lack of blood supply or from trauma. It results in a small, soft, non-functioning testicle.

19. *What are undescended testicles?*

In a male fetus, testicles develop in the lower abdominal cavity. During the seventh month of pregnancy, the testicles descend into the scrotal sac. If they fail to descend, they stay in the inguinal (groin) area of the lower abdominal cavity. The medical name for this condition is *cryptorchidism.*

20. *Do undescended testicles produce sperm?*

No, they do not. A man with undescended testicles is sterile.

21. *Why can't undescended testicles produce sperm?*

The temperature of the abdominal cavity is about 4 degrees warmer than the scrotal sac, and testicles will not function properly at this warmer temperature. Sperm are not produced. A man with bilateral undescended testicles is sterile.

22. *Can a man have only one undescended testicle?*

Yes. It is not uncommon for only one of the testicles to be undescended, with one testicle in the scrotum.

23. *If a man has one descended testicle, can he be fertile?*

Yes. The testicle in the scrotal sac should be able to produce sperm if everything else is normal. If this is the case, the undescended testicle should be removed to avoid development of cancer.

24. *Can undescended testicles be corrected?*

Surgery can be performed to move the testicles from the groin or lower abdomen and bring them into the scrotum. This is done by cutting the attachments around the testicle but not interfering with the blood supply.

25. *When is surgery performed?*

Surgery is performed during childhood, before a boy reaches school age. It should *not* be performed during infancy because testicles may descend on their own.

26. *Can testicles function normally in an adult after they are surgically corrected in childhood?*

They may, but there is a high percentage of men who are sterile after childhood surgery.

27. *What if undescended testicles are not corrected during childhood?*

There is a greater chance of developing cancer in the testicles as an adult if testicles are left in the groin or abdominal cavity. Any man with undescended testicles that were not corrected as a child should have them removed to prevent cancer from developing.

28. *What is testicular torsion?*

Torsion of the testicles is a condition in which the testicles twist on their ligaments, cutting off the blood supply. Twisting results in a marked swelling of the testicles; if left untreated, it may cause permanent damage.

29. *What causes testicular torsion?*

It is usually caused by a congenital defect in the ligaments that attach the testicle to the scrotum. Rarely, trauma to the testicles causes torsion.

30. *What is the treatment for testicular torsion?*

Immediate surgery to release the pressure and untwist the torsion is the treatment of choice. Stitches are placed between the testicles and the scrotal sac so the condition will not recur.

31. *What if surgery is not performed immediately?*

Occasionally, torsion of the testicles is misdiagnosed as an infection, and antibiotic treatment is given. If there is delay in performing surgery, testicles die and gradually shrivel to the size of a pea. If this happens, the testicle does not produce sperm.

32. *Does this result in sterility?*

Untreated testicular torsion results in sterility only if it occurs on *both* sides. One testicle will produce enough sperm for fertilization if its sperm production is normal.

33. *What is retrograde ejaculation?*

Retrograde ejaculation is the situation in which ejaculate (semen) goes backward into a man's bladder instead of going out of his penis.

34. *What causes retrograde ejaculation?*

It is caused by failure of the sphincter muscle (the muscle between the bladder and the urethra) to clamp down at the time of ejaculation. Ejaculation is a complex process that involves simultaneous excretion of semen and sperm from the vas deferens, seminal vesicles, prostate gland and periurethral glands. Interference with the nerve or blood supply to any of these organs can result in dysfunction of the ejaculatory mechanism.

35. *Who is most likely to develop retrograde ejaculation?*

It is most common in men who have diabetes. It may also occur after a man has surgery on his prostate gland or as a side effect of some medications.

36. *What can be done to treat retrograde ejaculation?*

It depends on what causes the problem. Medication to constrict the sphincter may help. If medication doesn't work, a catheter can be put in the bladder after intercourse or masturbation to retrieve sperm for use in artificial insemination.

37. *What is hypospadias?*

Hypospadias is a congenital birth defect of the penis. The urethral opening occurs on the *underside* of the penis rather than on the end. If this condition is not corrected, ejaculation would occur outside the vagina and sperm would not get into the cervical canal.

38. *What is the treatment for hypospadias?*

Surgery on the penis is necessary. It may have to be done in several stages if the opening is near the scrotal end of the penis. If surgery doesn't correct the condition, semen can be obtained by masturbation and used in artificial insemination.

39. *What abnormalities of the ductal system can cause infertility?*

A man can have a congenital absence of the vas deferens. The doctor will be aware of this if sperm are not found in the semen analysis. The absence of the vas deferens will be noticed during the physical exam. At this time, there is no known treatment for this condition.

Various infections, such as gonorrhea, chlamydia or mycoplasma, may cause a blockage of the ductal system. These obstructions are usually located at the junction of the epididymis and vas deferens.

40. *What is gonorrhea?*

Gonorrhea is a sexually transmitted disease caused by bacteria *Neisseria gonorrhea*. In a man, it causes inflammation of the urethra, resulting in a white, pus-filled discharge. In more severe cases, it can infect the prostate gland, vas deferens and epididymis and may cause permanent damage to these organs.

41. *How does gonorrhea affect fertility?*

Once the epididymis or vas deferens becomes in-flamed, scarring may result during the healing proc-ess. Scarring can cause blockage of the ductal system so sperm can't enter the ejaculate. It may also cause scarring of the penile urethra and partially obstruct the flow of urine from the bladder; this condition is called *urethral stricture.*

42. *What is the treatment for gonorrhea?*

Antibiotics, such as penicillin, tetracycline and erythromycin, are effective. The sooner gonorrhea is treated, the less likely it is to cause scarring.

43. *What are mycoplasma, ureaplasma and chlamydia infections?*

These are three organisms that may cause cervicitis and PID in a woman and urethritis, prostatitis and epididymitis in a man.

44. *What symptoms do they cause in a man?*

Men with mycoplasma, ureaplasma and chlamydia may not have any symptoms, or they may have a discharge from the penis. These organisms can cause non-specific urethritis (NSU), with burning during urination.

45. *How do mycoplasma, ureaplasma and chlamydia infections cause infertility?*

Mild infections may cause poor motility of sperm. If they cause cervicitis in a woman, it may result in poor cervical mucus. Mycoplasma, ureaplasma and chlamydial infections are found more frequently in infertile couples than in fertile couples, even if no symptoms are present. Your doctor should perform cultures for these organisms in cases of unexplained infertility.

46. *How are these organisms treated?*

Tetracycline is the treatment of choice. In cases of unexplained infertility, some doctors treat both partners with tetracycline, even though the cultures may prove negative. These organisms are often very difficult to culture. They may die in the process of obtaining them and transferring them to the lab for culture, resulting in a negative culture even when the organism is present.

47. *What is prostatitis?*

It is an infection and inflammation of the prostate gland that may be caused by one of many different organisms, such as chlamydia, gonorrhea and ureaplasma.

48. *What are the symptoms of prostatitis?*

Prostatitis may have no symptoms, or it may cause a discharge from the penis and a heavy-pressure feeling in the prostate gland below the bladder.

49. *How does prostatitis affect fertility?*

Part of the seminal fluid comes from the prostate gland. An infection will result in pus in the seminal fluid that is hostile to sperm survival. The semen analysis shows the presence of pus cells, poor sperm motility and possible clumping of sperm.

50. *How are infections of the prostate gland treated?*

Antibiotics usually cure an acute infection. It is not uncommon for some men to develop chronic prostatitis, which can be difficult to cure. Bacteria get into the deep glands of the prostate, which results in a chronic infection with pus cells in the semen even after long-term antibiotic treatment.

51. *Can anything be done in chronic prostatitis to improve the chance for pregnancy?*

Sperm-improvement techniques, such as sperm washing and swim-up techniques, can be used to clear the pus cells and debris from the semen. Sperm can then be used in artificial insemination.

52. *What are sperm washings and swim-up techniques?*

These are treatments used on sperm to help improve their ability to fertilize an egg. Semen is mixed and washed with a protein solution called Ham's solution then used in artificial insemination. See page 224 for additional information.

53. What is a swim-up technique?

In the swim-up technique, sperm are allowed to swim up a protein solution. The better, more mobile sperm are used in artificial insemination.

54. What is epididymitis?

Epididymitis is an infection of the epididymis, which is the place in a man's body where sperm mature and become capable of fertilizing an egg. Any infection that infects the prostate gland or urethra may also infect the epididymis.

55. How do infections of the epididymis affect fertility?

Infections of the epididymis may result in sperm that are not mature; blockage of the epididymal ducts is also a possibility. If blockage occurs, sperm are not present in the ejaculate and fructose is absent in the semen.

56. How are epididymal infections treated?

Antibiotics are used to treat the acute infection. If the acute infection is not treated, blockages of the ducts can result, and microsurgery may be necessary to open them.

57. *Can blockages of the ductal system be corrected?*

Most ductal-system blockages caused by infections occur between the epididymis and vas deferens. If the blockage is located in one or two areas, bypassing the blockage using microsurgical techniques may be possible. If there are numerous blockages through the entire vas deferens, treatment may be impossible.

58. *Can other types of illness affect fertility in a man?*

Because testicles are sensitive to heat, it is possible for any illness that causes a high fever to affect sperm production. It takes 72 days for sperm to mature, so an illness that affects sperm production may not be apparent for 2 to 3 months.

If a man has a low sperm count, it's important for the doctor to know if he has been sick during the previous 2 to 3 months. The sperm count should be repeated at a later time to see if the low count persists.

59. *Do other diseases affect fertility?*

Some autoimmune diseases, such as rheumatoid arthritis, ulcerative colitis and regional enteritis, may affect sperm production. This can be a result of the disease or the medication to treat it.

60. *How do hormone tests help determine the cause of male infertility?*

Evaluation of various hormone tests—FSH, LH, serum testosterone, prolactin, DHEAS and thyroid—enables the doctor to focus on the hypothalmus, pituitary, adrenal and thyroid glands as possible causes of male infertility.

61. *What is Kallman's Syndrome?*

Kallman's Syndrome is a lack of production of GNRH from the hypothalmus. Because there is no stimulation of the pituitary gland, FSH and LH are not produced, which results in no stimulation of sperm production from the testicles. Kallman's Syndrome is also called *hypogonadotropic hypogandism.*

62. *What are the symptoms of Kallman's Syndrome?*

Symptoms include a low or absent sperm count and anosmia (a person's inability to detect odors or loss of the sense of smell). Serum FSH and LH levels are also low.

63. *How is Kallman's Syndrome treated?*

It is treated with Pergonal injections (the same drug used to stimulate ovulation in a woman). This is very expensive because it costs over a $1,000 month for the Pergonal, and the drug must be given daily for *months* before sperm count improves.

64. *Is there any other treatment for Kallman's Syndrome?*

Recently, synthetic GNRH has been developed and may be the preferred treatment in the future.

65. *Can pituitary tumors occur in a man?*

A man may develop a pituitary gland adenoma or microadenoma, which causes an increase in prolactin secretion. An adenoma is a tumor greater than 10mm, and a microadenoma is less than 10mm. See pages 18 to 20.

66. *What problems does increased prolactin cause?*

An increase in prolactin will interfere with the secretion of FSH and LH, which results in poor sperm production in the testicles.

67. *What are the symptoms of a pituitary adenoma in a man?*

A man may develop a milky secretion from the breast (galactorrhea). Pituitary growths are usually discovered later in men than in women, resulting in larger tumors. The symptoms of headache, double vision or visual-field defects occur from a larger tumor pressing on the optic nerve. A gradual loss of sexual function, such as impotence and loss of sexual desire, may also be present.

68. *How are pituitary tumors treated in a man?*

If the pituitary growth is very small, bromocryptine (Parlodel) can be used to shrink the tumor. If the tumor is large, a combination of Parlodel and surgical removal may be necessary.

69. *How is clomiphene citrate (Clomid) used in treating male infertility?*

Clomiphene citrate is commonly used in a woman to stimulate ovulation. It is also used in a man to stimulate sperm production. When a man takes the drug, he takes it daily throughout the month, rather than 5 days each month as a woman does.

70. *How does clomiphene citrate work?*

It stimulates FSH and LH production; the increase in FSH and LH stimulates the seminiferous tubules to produce more sperm and stimulates Leydig cells to increase their production of testosterone.

71. *How long does it take to find out if clomiphene citrate is effective?*

It may take several months to see if there is improvement in the semen analysis. The time interval from beginning sperm production in the testicles to their appearance in the ejaculate is 72 days, so it will require 2 to 3 months as a minimum to see if there is improvement in sperm production.

72. *Are all infertile men candidates for clomiphene citrate?*

No. It is usually given to men who do not have a varicocele but do have low sperm counts and poor motility. Studies of clomiphene citrate treatment have been analyzed with mixed results. Some men experience improved sperm counts; others do not. If a varicocele is present, it is usually treated before the drug is prescribed because of the documented success of spermatic-vein ligation in treating infertility.

73. *What are side effects when clomiphene citrate is taken by a man?*

Hot flashes and visual disturbances have been reported with high doses. A man usually tolerates the drug fairly well. A positive side effect is an increase in a man's sex drive along with an increase in the frequency of sexual intercourse.

74. *I've heard about testosterone rebound. What is this?*

This is a form of hormonal therapy that was used years ago. It involves giving a low dose of testosterone to infertile men. Testosterone temporarily makes the sperm count lower because it decreases the production of FSH and LH. When testosterone is stopped, there is a marked rise in FSH and LH secretion, hopefully with a stimulation of sperm production.

75. *Why isn't testosterone rebound used more frequently?*

The use of clomiphene citrate has generally replaced its use, but testosterone rebound is still tried in some men. Both clomiphene citrate and testosterone rebound attempt to increase FSH and LH production. Clomiphene citrate is easier to take, and results are more promising. Some men were found to be less fertile after testosterone rebound therapy.

76. *What is the role of HCG in male infertility?*

HCG is similar to LH; it is used in men and has an effect on the testicles similar to clomiphene citrate. The disadvantage of HCG is that it is given by injection and has to be given at least 3 times a week for several months. Use of clomiphene citrate has almost replaced its use.

77. *What is Klinefelter's Syndrome?*

Klinefelter's Syndrome is a chromosomal abnormality; a man is born with an XXY sex chromosome arrangement, rather than the normal male XY. The female comparison to this syndrome is Turner's Syndrome. See pages 162 to 164.

78. *What are the symptoms of Klinefelter's Syndrome?*

Men with Klinefelter's Syndrome have poorly developed genitals, gynecomastia (increase in breast size) and scarring in the seminiferous tubules of the testicles. Most men with Klinefelter's Syndrome do not produce sperm; they are sterile.

79. *How is Klinefelter's Syndrome diagnosed?*

FSH in the blood is usually elevated, and a testicular biopsy will show scarring of the seminiferous tubules. A chromosome study can be done for definite diagnosis.

80. *Is there treatment for Klinefelter's Syndrome?*

There is no treatment.

81. *What is impotence?*

Impotence is the inability of a man to have an erection and/or ejaculation.

82. *What are the causes of impotence?*

The causes of impotence are usually divided into two categories—emotional and physical.

83. *What is emotional impotence?*

Emotional impotence in infertile couples is common; don't be alarmed if it occurs. The stress of trying to become pregnant is the most common factor. Having timed intercourse according to a schedule, rather than when you desire, may also result in impotence.

Impotence may occur during an infertility investigation when a post-coital test is scheduled. A request to perform intercourse is often made at an unusual hour (very early in the morning), which puts undue pressure on the man, who is unable to have an erection.

You may be embarrassed to tell your doctor about this problem, and it may be one reason for a poor post-coital test. A doctor who treats infertile couples is usually very understanding of this condition, so don't be embarrassed to discuss it with him.

84. *Are there other causes of emotional impotence?*

Any stressful situation in a man's life, such as job-related stress or a recent death in the family, may result in impotence.

85. *How is emotional impotence treated?*

If you believe the stress of infertility is the cause, take a break from trying to conceive. If stress is related to your husband's job or other factors, impotence may only be temporary. Try to discover the cause, discuss it and work out any problems. Professional counseling may be necessary.

86. *What are the causes of physical impotence?*

Physical impotence is caused by many different factors. Men with diabetes occasionally have nerve damage to the genital organs; this can result in impotence. Previous prostate-gland surgery may also result in impotence.

87. *What can be done for physical impotence?*

If treating the basic disease causing the impotence does not help the impotence, the surgical insertion of a penile implant to maintain an erect penis may be a solution.

88. *Can medication cause impotence?*

Medication, such as tranquilizers, anti-depressants, antihistamines and anti-hypertensives, may cause impotence as a side effect. If your husband takes any medication and impotence occurs, have him check with his doctor to see if the medication is a possible cause.

89. *Do thyroid abnormalities cause male infertility?*

Abnormal thyroid production can cause poor sperm production in a man. If thyroid tests are abnormal, appropriate medication can be prescribed.

90. *What if thyroid tests are normal?*

Years ago, every man with an abnormal semen analysis was treated with thyroid medication to try to improve his semen analysis—even if he had normal thyroid function. Some of these men did impregnate their wives, but in critical evaluation of the studies performed, thyroid medication was found *not* to be of benefit. It was believed the women who became pregnant would have conceived even if the husband had not taken the medication. Today, thyroid medication is not recommended unless a man's thyroid tests are abnormal.

10

What Is Unexplained Infertility?

Unexplained infertility is not well-understood, even by fertility specialists. When an infertility investigation is finished and nothing is found, researchers believe the reason for infertility may be in the immune system.

1. *What is "unexplained infertility"?*

It is infertility that cannot be explained with our present technical knowledge. There may be a reason for the infertility, but we just don't know it. Researchers believe a large percentage of unexplained infertility is related to immunolgic infertility and the immune system.

2. *What does immunologic mean?*

Immunologic refers to the body's immune system—it is a complicated system that enables the body to fight off foreign substances and certain diseases. As a child, when you received immunizations against diseases, such as polio, rubella, diphtheria, whooping cough tetanus, you were given an injection of a substance called an antigen. The antigen stimulated the formation of antibodies, which prevented you from becoming ill from these diseases. Your immune system produced the antibodies.

3. *What organs in the body make up the immune system?*

The immune system is made up of the lymphoid tissue—the spleen, lymph nodes, bone marrow, plasma cells and the leukocytes (white blood cells in the bloodstream). This system is responsible for production of antibodies and allergic reactions.

4. *What is an antigen?*

An *antigen* is a protein or proteinlike substance that stimulates the immune system to produce antibodies. An *antibody* produced by a specific antigen remains in your system to react with that antigen if it is exposed to it again.

5. *How does the immune system work?*

When an immunization against a disease, such as measles, is given, the vaccine (an antigen similar to the actual virus but which doesn't cause illness) is the protein substance that stimulates production of an antibody. The antibody remains in your bloodstream indefinitely. If it is challenged by another antigen (such as the measles virus), the antibody reacts with the antigen so you don't become ill.

The immune system can also cause allergic reactions

to a particular drug or food. Hives or a rash are the end results of the antigen (the drug or food) and antibody reaction.

Your immune system may also reject foreign substances, such as an organ transplant. Some diseases result from attacking our own body tissues, such as rheumatoid arthritis, lupus erythematosus and some forms of diabetes. These diseases are called *auto-immune diseases*.

6. *How does the immune system relate to infertility?*

The antigen-antibody reaction is the basis for *immunologic infertility;* a woman is allergic to a man's sperm or semen. Sperm and semen are foreign substances in a woman's body, so one might expect all women to develop antibodies to sperm. For reasons we don't fully understand, most women do *not* develop antibodies to sperm—only 3% of all *infertile* women are allergic to sperm. These women can form antibodies to all sperm or just their husband's sperm.

7. *How is immunologic infertility diagnosed?*

A post-coital test may be the first indication of an allergy to sperm. The sperm present in a post-coital test do not move; if they do move, they are very sluggish. This may indicate an allergic reaction in which your mucus kills sperm. If this is the case, a cervical-mucus-sperm-penetration assay may be recommended.

8. *What is a cervical-mucus-sperm-penetration assay?*

It is a method of determining the compatibility between your cervical mucus and sperm. Mucus obtained from you at midcycle and sperm from your husband and sperm from a known-fertile man are studied together.

The penetration of the two different sperm samples into the mucus is checked. If your mucus does not react well with either specimen, you are checked for sperm antibodies in your mucus and blood. It's possible to be incompatible with only your husband's sperm.

In the same manner, your husband's sperm can be checked for penetration into your mucus and that of a known-fertile woman. Depending on the results of these tests, one can conclude if you or your husband are allergic to all sperm or mucus, or just each other's.

9. *Can a man be allergic to his own sperm?*

It is possible for a man to develop an allergy to his own sperm, often after a vasectomy. We believe this is from the inability of sperm to escape from the testicles and epididymis. When sperm remains in the testicles and epididymis, it enables the body to develop antibodies against the sperm. This is an important consideration if a man is considering vasectomy reversal. Sperm allergies can also develop for other reasons that we do not yet fully understand.

10. *How is male sperm allergy diagnosed?*

The semen analysis may show tail-to-tail or head-to-head agglutination (clumping together). If agglutination is present, it usually indicates sperm allergy. But it does not have to be present for sperm allergy to exist.

11. *Are there anti-sperm-antibody tests available to check for sperm allergy?*

Yes. Men and women can have their blood checked for antibodies against sperm. In addition, seminal fluid in a man and cervical mucus in a woman can be checked for antibodies against sperm.

12. *Who should be checked for anti-sperm antibodies?*

Men with unexplained infertility or sperm agglutination on a semen analysis or men who are contemplating a vasectomy reversal should have their anti-sperm-antibody level checked. A man with an increase in non-motile sperm in a semen analysis and a man whose wife has a poor post-coital test or poor penetration on a cervical-mucus-sperm-penetration test should also consider antibody testing. Women with unexplained infertility and sperm immobilization on a post-coital test should be checked for antibodies.

13. *How reliable are these tests?*

These tests are *not* 100% accurate. Infertile couples may have antibodies present, but many fertile couples also have antibodies. These tests are helpful in trying to prescribe treatment for this very difficult, puzzling aspect of infertility.

14. *What is the hamster-egg-penetration assay?*

This is a relatively new test that determines the ability of the sperm to penetrate and fertilize an egg once the sperm reach the site of fertilization. The test is believed to be a good correlation with the ability of the man being tested to impregnate his wife. It is being used in cases of unexplained infertility and in a few other areas of infertility.

15. *How is the hamster-egg-penetration assay performed?*

Hamsters are superovulated with drugs that induce ovulation. Twenty to 25 hamster eggs are mixed with human sperm and incubated for a certain length of time. Eggs are checked to see if sperm have penetrated them.

16. *What kind of results can we expect?*

A normal result shows at least 20 to 25% of the eggs have been penetrated by sperm. If none of the eggs have been penetrated, it probably indicates sperm are incapable of fertilization.

17. *When should the hamster-egg-penetration assay be performed?*

The test is useful in unexplained infertility, in men with minor semen defects, in men with varicoceles but normal semen qualities, and in couples who are contemplating in-vitro fertilization. A man must have at least 5 million sperm/cc to have the test performed.

18. *Is there any treatment for an abnormal hamster-egg-penetration assay?*

There is no known treatment at this time if sperm do not show penetration. Researchers are studying treatment of sperm with different protein solutions, such as in sperm washings, to try to improve the results of a penetration assay.

19. *How expensive is the hamster-egg-penetration assay?*

It is one of the more expensive infertility tests because of the work involved in performing the test and the cost of the hamsters. The cost varies, depending on where the test is performed, but it generally costs about $300. The test is only available in specialized infertility laboratories at this time.

20. *How can immunologic infertility be treated?*

Treating immunologic infertility is one of the most difficult aspects of infertility. Many treatments are based on hunch rather than scientific knowledge. If either you or your husband is allergic to sperm, medication to decrease the allergic response and to reduce the production of antibodies to sperm may be tried.

21. *Which medications reduce antibody production?*

Medications similar to those used to suppress the immune system in organ-transplant patients are too powerful and have too many side effects to be used in infertility. A cortisone preparation, such as prednisone or dexamethasone, is usually prescribed.

Cortisone medications have side effects, such as ulcers, diabetes, weight gain, osteoporosis and psychosis; these limit their use in large doses. Men and women found to be allergic to sperm can be put on cortisone medication if they understand the possible side effects. Treatment with cortisone has been successful in selected patients. Condom therapy can be used if you are allergic to your husband's sperm.

22. *What is condom therapy?*

In condom therapy, the man uses a condom during intercourse to keep sperm from coming in contact with mucus. This decreases your exposure to sperm and decreases your production of antibodies against the sperm. Condom therapy is used continuously for 6 months, then the condom is omitted at midcycle to try to conceive.

23. *How successful is condom therapy?*

After 6 months of condom therapy, the post-coital test may show active sperm in the cervical mucus. Condom therapy has worked for many couples, but it is not the answer to immunologic infertility.

Some couples become frustrated because during the

6 months of using condoms there is no chance of becoming pregnant. Some doctors feel the success rate is not any greater if you use condom therapy.

24. *What else can be done for immunologic and unexplained infertility?*

Performing artificial insemination with the husband's sperm (AIH) provides the best results. If you don't conceive using your husband's semen, various techniques to improve the sperm's qualities may be tried to improve the chance for pregnancy.

25. *What are sperm-improvement techniques?*

These are techniques in which sperm are treated in a laboratory to try to improve their quality before placing them in the woman by AIH. The purpose of the technique is to improve sperm motility and the concentration of normal-looking, active sperm and to increase the penetrating capacity of the sperm.

26. *How is this done?*

This is done by various techniques, including *sperm washings* and *swim-up techniques*.

27. *What are sperm washings, and what do they accomplish?*

Sperm are separated from the seminal fluid and "washed" in an artificial protein solution, called Ham's medium, that improves the sperm's motility, longevity and penetrating capacity. Washing has been shown to improve sperm function in preparation for cervical or intrauterine inseminations and to "wash off" antibodies that may be present in the semen. After the washings, sperm are artificially inseminated into the woman.

28. *Who are candidates for sperm washings?*

In men with sperm antibodies, washings remove antigen and antibodies in the semen. This technique is also used in couples with poor cervical-mucus-sperm interaction, indicating an immunologic cause for infertility.

The technique of sperm washings is being used in more cases of unexplained infertility in which the infertility evaluation is normal. It is also used in cases of decreased sperm motility not associated with a varicocele and in cases of retrograde ejaculation. Sperm washings are also used to treat sperm prior to in-vitro fertilization.

29. *How successful is the technique of sperm washings?*

Preliminary studies from large clinics show a 25 to 45% pregnancy rate following six cycles of artificial insemination using sperm washings and LH-timed inseminations. These tests were done in women who were previously infertile, so the technique shows some hope.

30. *What is the swim-up technique to improve sperm quality?*

This technique is used for men who have a large amount of debris, such as pus cells, in their semen. Washed sperm are placed in a special protein solution and allowed to swim up the top of the solution, leaving most of the debris behind. The sperm that were able to swim up are the most active, normal sperm; they are then concentrated and used in artificial insemination.

31. *Can all doctors perform these sperm-improvement techniques?*

These techniques are relatively new and require special equipment, so they may not be available by most doctors who treat infertile patients. These techniques are usually performed in large infertility clinics.

It may be possible to have sperm washings performed at an infertility laboratory, then take the specimen to your own doctor for insemination. If these techniques prove successful, they should become more accessible in the future.

11

When Should We Consider Artificial Insemination?

When you and your husband have undergone all the tests and have your final results, you may want to consider an artificial method of conceiving a pregnancy. One of the most-discussed and well-known methods is artificial insemination. As a couple, this may be one alternative to consider.

1. *What is artificial insemination?*

Artificial insemination is a procedure in which semen from a man is artificially placed into the cervical canal or uterus of a woman for the purpose of conception.

2. *What methods of artificial insemination are there?*

There are two methods of artificial insemination:
1. Semen from your husband is used. This is called *artificial insemination by the husband* or *AIH.*
2. Semen from a man other than your husband is used; it is usually obtained from a man unknown to you. This is called *artificial insemination by donor* or *AID.*

3. *Why is artificial insemination from the husband (AIH) recommended?*

There are several reasons why this method of artificial insemination is performed. It is most commonly performed when the husband has a borderline semen analysis with a low-sperm count (below 20 million) and poor sperm motility. Results of the post-coital test reveal few, if any, active sperm in the cervical mucus. Many dead sperm may be present in the cervical mucus.

AIH allows the doctor to place sperm into the cervical canal or uterine cavity to give sperm a greater chance to reach the Fallopian tube. In some cases, it may be helpful to use a split ejaculate.

4. *What is a split ejaculate?*

With a split-ejaculate specimen, semen is obtained in two containers. The first part of the ejaculate is collected in one container and the second part in another.

5. *What is the purpose of using a split ejaculate?*

Usually the first part of the ejaculate contains a much higher concentration of sperm than the second part. The second part is nearly all seminal fluid.

Using the first part in artificial insemination may give a greater concentration of sperm in the mucus and improve chances for success. This is especially true in men with a high volume of seminal fluid (greater than 5cc).

If this technique is used, sperm counts in each part of the ejaculate are checked to make sure there is a higher concentration of sperm in the first part of the specimen. Occasionally, the second part is better. If there is no significant difference in the two parts, split-ejaculate insemination has no advantage.

6. *Is artificial insemination used in immunologic infertility?*

AIH can be tried when sperm and mucus are incompatible and mucus may immobilize the sperm. Semen may be placed directly into the uterus to bypass the cervical mucus. This is done very carefully because if semen escapes out of the uterus, through the Fallopian tubes into the abdominal cavity, it can cause severe abdominal pain.

Sperm washings have been performed prior to use in artificial insemination, with an improved rate of success. The purpose of the washings is to remove antibodies that may be present and to improve the sperm's motility. See page 224.

7. *Is artificial insemination indicated in cases of unexplained infertility?*

This is an area that is being explored. It's similar to AIH use in immunologic infertility with sperm washings, and it is being tried in cases of unexplained infertility. Further studies must be performed before this can be recommended without question.

8. *What are other indications for AIH?*

Another indication for AIH would be when a couple's intercourse technique does not allow sperm to enter the vagina or cervix. Examples of this problem include a markedly obese couple who has problems with the penis entering the vagina during intercourse or the case of a man with retrograde ejaculation whose semen goes into his bladder rather than out through his penis. Artificial insemination eliminates these obstacles.

9. *Is AIH more successful than normal intercourse?*

If there is a normal post-coital test, there is no evidence artificial insemination improves your chance of pregnancy. Performing sperm washings may be an exception, but it may be too early to conclude this without further research.

10. *What is artificial insemination by donor (AID)?*

AID, not to be confused with AIDS (Acquired Immune Deficiency Syndrome), inseminates the wife with sperm from a donor other than the husband. The donor is usually unknown to the couple.

11. *When is AID recommended?*

It is recommended when the husband is sterile or when his sperm count is so low that pregnancy is believed to be impossible.

12. *Where does the doctor find sperm to use?*

Freshly obtained semen from a man with a normal semen analysis can be used. This man is usually very accessible to the doctor's office where insemination is performed. In places with medical schools, medical-school students have typically been the largest source of donors. Frozen sperm from a sperm bank can also be used.

13. *What are sperm banks?*

Sperm banks were established for the purpose of storing a man's sperm and also to create a pool of donors for use in artificial insemination. Occasionally, large infertility clinics may have their own sperm banks.

14. *How is sperm stored in a sperm bank?*

After semen is mixed with glycerol to help sperm survive, it is frozen by liquid nitrogen, then stored until it is needed. Sperm can be kept frozen for years and still survive. Semen can be shipped anywhere in the country, using liquid nitrogen or dry ice, then thawed in the doctor's office when it is needed.

15. *How well does sperm survive the freezing process?*

A certain percentage of sperm don't survive. Sperm from men with a borderline semen analysis do not freeze well, so sperm are not usually stored for later insemination. For semen to be used after it is frozen, sperm count and motility must be in the normal range.

16. *Is it better to use fresh or frozen sperm when performing AID?*

There are pros and cons of using each type. A certain percentage of sperm do not survive the freezing process, so it's usually better to use fresh semen. Studies comparing the two have shown better results from fresh semen. A larger selection of donors is usually available using frozen sperm from large sperm banks.

17. *Is it possible to get a venereal disease or Acquired Immune Deficiency Syndrome (AIDS) from donor insemination?*

Yes, this is possible. Donors are usually screened for sexually transmitted diseases, but this does not guarantee they haven't contracted a venereal disease after being screened. This has become more of a concern because of publicity about AIDS. The AIDS virus can be transmitted in semen; as a result, some artificial-insemination clinics have switched from fresh to frozen sperm to allow better control over possible disease in donors.

18. *Will a woman receiving AID know the identity of the donor?*

This is kept strictly confidential to avoid problems regarding paternity responsibility or other problems that may arise in the future.

19. *Does the donor know who is receiving his sperm?*

No. For the same reasons as mentioned above, it is kept strictly confidential.

20. *Is it wise to use a friend or relative as a donor?*

It is not wise to use a friend or relative. Even though a friend or relative may give consent and understand he has no claim on the child, there is no guarantee that several years after the insemination he won't try to claim paternal responsibility.

21. *How does the doctor select his donors?*

Donors are usually screened for above-average intelligence, freedom from communicable and venereal diseases, and no family history of genetic abnormalities.

22. *Is the donor the same race as the husband?*

Yes.

23. *If the husband and wife are of a minority race, is it possible to find a suitable donor?*

It depends on the source of donors. If your doctor has a large source, it should be possible. Minority-race donors are usually available from large sperm banks using frozen sperm.

24. *Is it possible to match the husband's characteristics, such as skin color, hair color, eye color and nationality, to that of the donor?*

This is done as much as possible; it depends on the availability of donors. Using frozen sperm from a large sperm bank may provide a better selection of donors to obtain all the characteristics desired.

25. *Is donor insemination expensive?*

It is more expensive than AIH. In addition to the usual expense of performing the insemination, the donor or sperm bank must be paid for the semen. This may be an additional $50 to $150 per insemination, depending on how much the doctor has to pay for the semen.

26. *Do some couples have difficulty accepting donor insemination?*

Yes; you should thoroughly discuss it between yourselves and with your doctor *before* agreeing to donor insemination. The husband is not the genetic father, so there is a possibility he may feel uninvolved in your pregnancy or raising the child.

27. *What are the legalities of AID?*

All the legal ramifications of artificial insemination by donor have not been totally resolved. In most states, the birth certificate is filled out with the husband as the genetic father of the baby. In some states, the law may require the father to legally adopt a child conceived by AID. The couple having the child must take full responsibility for the outcome of the pregnancy, even if the child is born with birth defects.

28. *Can the husband's semen be mixed with the donor's?*

This is done occasionally.

29. *Why would a mixed insemination be done?*

Occasionally, if a husband has some sperm in his semen specimen, a couple will request a mixed insemination to allow the husband the chance of being the father of the pregnancy. If pregnancy does occur with a mixed insemination, it would be impossible to know who the father is without a paternity investigation after the child's birth.

30. *Is it harmful to mix the donor's and husband's semen?*

The reason for AID is the poor quality of the husband's semen; mixing it with good donor semen may make the resulting semen less effective in achieving pregnancy.

31. *How is the semen specimen obtained when using the husband's sperm?*

The man is asked to masturbate into a sterile container. This can be done in the doctor's office or at home just before your appointment for the insemination. If the specimen is collected at home, the woman immediately brings it to the doctor's office. It's best to have the insemination performed within 1 hour of obtaining the specimen.

32. *How is the semen specimen obtained in donor inseminations?*

If fresh-donor insemination is used, the donor usually leaves the specimen just before the woman's appointment. The specimen is obtained by masturbation, similar to obtaining the specimen for AIH. It is collected in a different part of the office or building, so the donor and the recipient do not see each other. If a frozen specimen is used, it is usually kept frozen until just before the specimen is used.

33. *How is artificial insemination performed?*

After placing a speculum into your vagina, semen is placed into the cervical canal or uterus with a small catheter or tube. Some doctors use a cervical cap or diaphragm to keep semen in contact with the cervix after the insemination is performed.

You remain on the examination table for about 20 minutes following the insemination, then you may leave to go about your normal activities. If a cervical cap or diaphragm was used, it is removed by you after a few hours.

34. *Is artificial insemination painful?*

Usually, artificial insemination is no more uncomfortable than having a pelvic examination. Occasionally, a slight cramp is felt when the semen is placed into the cervical canal.

If semen is placed into the uterus and escapes into the abdominal cavity by going out the Fallopian tubes, severe abdominal pain may be experienced, but this is rare. Pain is caused by the seminal fluid (not sperm) causing a severe reaction with the peritoneum (the lining around the intestines, uterus, tubes and ovaries). The pain may last for a few hours, then gradually it goes away.

35. *When in my menstrual cycle is artificial insemination performed?*

Artificial insemination is performed as close to ovulation as possible. This is usually determined by having you take your basal body temperature for a period of time before artificial insemination to help schedule the timed inseminations.

Continue taking your BBT while undergoing the procedure to schedule future inseminations if you do not become pregnant. Using one of the ovulation-predictor tests has helped with timing of artificial insemination.

36. *How many inseminations are done each month?*

The number of inseminations performed each month depends on the regularity of your menstrual cycle. If your cycle is regular, only one or two inseminations per cycle may be done. If it is irregular, more will have to be performed so ovulation is not missed.

Sperm can live for 48 to 72 hours, so inseminations are usually done every other day, but they may be done daily or every third day. Using one of the ovulation-predictor tests while undergoing artificial insemination may reduce the number of inseminations needed each month to one or two.

37. *What if I have very irregular cycles and need artificial insemination?*

If you have irregular cycles, one of the ovulation-inducing drugs, such as Clomid, can be used and artificial insemination scheduled accordingly.

12

Can Past Methods of Birth Control Affect Fertility?

Some women blame the methods they used for birth control on their problems with fertility. In some cases, past methods of birth control do contribute to fertility problems, but this is by no means the case for every woman. Don't automatically blame yourself or the method of birth control you used if you are having a fertility problem. This section should help you put your mind to rest regarding "blame."

1. *What is contraception?*

It is the prevention of conception or pregnancy and is often called *birth control*.

2. *What is a contraceptive?*

A contraceptive is any device or medication used to prevent conception.

3. *What are the different methods of birth control?*

We usually speak of permanent and non-permanent methods of birth control. *Permanent methods* are permanent and include vasectomy in men and tubal sterilization and hysterectomies in women. *Non-permanent methods* are temporary and include IUD, diaphragm, foam, condoms, vaginal suppositories and sponges, cervical caps and birth-control pills. Other methods use some variation of the rhythm method, such as temperature regulation and checking cervical mucus; this is called *natural family planning.*

4. *What are birth-control pills?*

The birth-control pill contains synthetic derivatives of estrogen and progesterone in various quantities. Although the technical name for the birth-control pill is *oral contraceptive,* we often call it "the pill."

5. *Is the combination of estrogen and progesterone the only pill there is?*

No, there is also a pill that contains only progesterone. It is taken every day rather than 3 weeks on, 1 week off, as the combination pill is taken.

6. *Are there side effects with the progesterone-only pill?*

Yes. It can cause irregular periods, and it has a higher pregnancy rate (about 4%) than the combination pill. It is not commonly used.

7. *When is the progesterone-only pill used?*

It is usually given to women who can't take estrogen but who prefer the pill to other methods of birth control.

8. *How does the birth-control pill work?*

It works by stopping ovulation. The pill prevents the egg from being released from the ovary by preventing release of FSH and LH from the pituitary gland. Without FSH and LH stimulation, the ovaries do not develop eggs, and ovulation does not occur.

9. *After a woman discontinues the pill, is it harder to become pregnant?*

In most cases, the pill has no effect. A small percentage of women (about 1%) who stop taking the pill do not resume ovulation or menstruation for 6 to 12 months. In this case, it is impossible to become pregnant during this time. This condition is called *post-pill amenorrhea.*

10. *Does this affect some women more than others?*

Yes. It is more common in women who had irregular periods before taking the pill than in women who had regular periods.

11. *What are irregular periods?*

Most women are on a regular 28-to-32-day menstrual cycle. From the first day of one period to the first day of another period is 28 to 32 days. Some women menstruate only every 6 to 12 weeks. It is with these women that post-pill amenorrhea is more common.

12. *Is it normal to have irregular periods when the pill is discontinued?*

Most women resume their periods in a pattern similar to the one they had before they took the pill. When the pill is stopped, it is normal for the first period to be 7 to 10 days "late." It is not unusual if the first few periods off the pill are slightly irregular. If this happens, it usually lasts only for a few months.

13. *How can post-pill amenorrhea be treated?*

Often it resolves without treatment. If you are anxious to try for pregnancy, an ovulation-inducing drug can be used.

14. *How long should I be off the pill before trying to become pregnant?*

Stop the pill at least 3 months before trying to become pregnant. Early reports indicated a higher miscarriage rate if you become pregnant in the first few cycles off the pill. Later studies showed this was untrue, but the recommendation still is advised. It allows your cycles to become normal, making it easier to predict a due date when you become pregnant. It also allows the hormones from the pill to get out of your system.

15. *What if I accidentally become pregnant before 3 months is up?*

This shouldn't be a great concern. If the pregnancy proceeds normally, there should be no greater risk of abnormalities than there would be if you conceived at a later time.

16. *What should be done for birth control during the first 3 months off the pill?*

A barrier-method of birth control, such as a diaphragm, foam or condoms, is recommended for this short interval.

17. *Are some women more fertile after taking the pill?*

This used to be a belief, but it is untrue.

18. *Are multiple pregnancies more common after taking the pill?*

No, they are not.

19. *Can I become pregnant while taking the pill?*

If you take the pill correctly, the pregnancy rate is about 0.5%—1 in 200 women who are on the pill may become pregnant while taking it. Of course, if you forget to take your pills regularly, the pregnancy rate is higher. Some antibiotics also render birth-control pills less effective. Be sure to advise your doctor you take birth-control pills when you need an antibiotic.

20. *What if I believe I'm pregnant while taking the pill?*

If you feel you may be pregnant while taking the pill, see your doctor immediately.

21. *What is an IUD?*

An IUD is an intrauterine device inserted into the uterus to prevent pregnancy. Years ago, IUDs were made of metal. Today, IUDs are plastic or plastic wrapped with a small amount of copper. Lippie's Loop, Progestasert, Copper-7 and Tatum-T are used most often today.

22. *How does an IUD work?*

It works by creating a hostile environment in the uterine lining that prevents implantation of a fertilized egg. It may also interfere with the movement of the tubes, and this prevents fertilization. Some doctors believe the action of an IUD is similar to an early miscarriage.

23. *Can an IUD cause infertility problems?*

Definitely! A woman with an IUD is 4 to 9 times more likely to develop pelvic inflammatory disease (PID) than a woman who does not have an IUD. This can result in scarring around the Fallopian tubes or blocked Fallopian tubes.

24. *Does an IUD increase my chances of contracting a sexually transmitted disease?*

No, it does not. Most infections you get with an IUD

are not caused by the IUD. It is possible to get a sexually transmitted disease, such as gonorrhea or chlamydia, with or without an IUD. But it appears that if an IUD is in place, an infection may be *more severe*, with a greater chance of causing PID, which may result in damage to the Fallopian tubes.

25. *Is there a higher incidence of tubal pregnancies in women who use IUDs?*

Yes, there is. If you get pelvic inflammatory disease, it will increase your chances of a tubal pregnancy. An IUD prevents intrauterine pregnancies but not tubal pregnancies. If you become pregnant with an IUD in place, there's always the possibility of a tubal pregnancy.

26. *What is the Dalkon shield?*

The Dalkon shield is an IUD that has recently received a lot of attention because of the many medical-legal problems and lawsuits over its use.

27. *What was wrong with the Dalkon shield?*

Its biggest problem was it contained a multifilament string (many strands of string made up a single strand), which enabled bacteria to grow between the filaments. This resulted in a greater risk of infection. The Dalkon shield is no longer available.

28. *Do other IUDs contain a multifilament string?*

No, they do not. They all contain a monofilament (single-strand) string.

29. *Will IUDs be available in the future?*

Many companies have stopped production and re-called all unused IUDs. The cost of defending lawsuits over use of IUDs and the cost of product-liability insurance has become astronomical. This will probably affect all IUDs in the near future, and they may not be available.

30. *What is a diaphragm?*

A diaphragm is a molded rubber cap that fits over the cervix. It is inserted into the vagina before intercourse, along with a contraceptive jelly, to keep sperm from entering the cervix and uterus.

31. *What does the contraceptive jelly do?*

It is spermicidal; it kills sperm.

32. *Does using a diaphragm have any bearing on future fertility?*

No, it has no effect on fertility. But it is interesting to note that women who use diaphragms are twice as likely to develop bladder infections than women who do not use them.

33. *What are foams, suppositories, creams, jellies and sponges?*

They are contraceptives that are inserted into the vagina before intercourse to prevent pregnancy.

34. *How do these contraceptives work?*

They contain an ingredient that kills sperm. It is basically the same ingredient but present in different forms.

35. *Are there side effects using these contraceptives?*

Occasionally they cause local irritation or allergic reaction in the vagina or on the penis.

36. *Do they affect future fertility?*

There is no known problem with future childbearing when these contraceptives are used.

37. *What is a condom?*

It is a rubber sheath that is placed over a man's erect penis just before intercourse to keep sperm from entering the vagina.

38. *Does it affect future fertility?*

No. In fact, it reduces the risk of passing on or getting a sexually transmitted disease if used with intercourse on a regular basis.

39. *What is a tubal ligation?*

It is a procedure in which Fallopian tubes are tied, cut, burned or clipped to prevent future pregnancies. It is considered a permanent, non-reversible procedure.

40. *How is tubal ligation performed?*

It can be performed in many different ways. The most common way is to have it done by laparoscopy. It may also be done following the birth of a baby or with a Cesarean section.

41. *Once tubes are "tied," is it possible to "untie" them?*

It is possible, but it depends on the type of sterilization procedure performed. Some sterilization procedures may remove part of the tube, including the fimbria. If the fimbria are removed, there is *no* chance for a reversal procedure. Occasionally, during a C-section or an abdominal operation, the Fallopian tube is completely removed or buried in the uterus. If this is the case, there is no chance for reversal.

If too much of the tube was cauterized at the time of the sterilization procedure, there is no chance for reversal. The best chance of having a tubal reversal performed is when only a small, midportion of the tube is removed, cauterized or clipped or when a ring is placed over the middle of the tube.

42. *What is the procedure called to untie or reunite the tubes?*

It is called *tubal-reversal surgery* or *tubal anastamosis* (reconnecting the tubes).

43. *How is this surgery performed?*

It is major surgery, with a full abdominal incision. Scar tissue where tubes were tied or cauterized is removed, then the ends of the tubes are reconnected. It is relatively easy to do a tubal sterilization but very difficult to put the tubes back together.

44. *How is tubal-reversal surgery usually done?*

Today, it is usually performed using microsurgical techniques.

45. *How long is hospitalization and recovery?*

It requires 3 to 5 days of hospitalization and 2 to 6 weeks to fully recover.

46. *What is microsurgery?*

Microsurgery uses an operating microscope or special glasses to magnify Fallopian tubes. This enables the surgeon to use very fine stitches to reconnect tubes. Fine stitches result in less scarring and a better chance for the tubes to be open after surgery.

47. *What should be done before considering a tubal reversal?*

Your past records should be reviewed to see what type of sterilization procedure was performed. If a fimbriectomy was performed or the entire tube was removed, it is impossible to have a reversal. A hysterosalpingogram may be necessary to see how much tube is still attached to the uterus. See page 112.

48. *What is a fimbriectomy?*

It is a type of tubal ligation in which the part of the tube closest to the ovary is removed. This part of the tube contains the fimbria that are responsible for picking up the eggs from the ovary at the time of ovulation. Without the fimbria, it is impossible to get pregnant the natural way.

49. *What happens if I have had a fimbriectomy?*

If you have had this type of tubal ligation, you are not a candidate for tubal-reversal surgery. However, you may be a candidate for in-vitro fertilization because the Fallopian tubes can be bypassed, with conception occurring outside the body. Then the fertilized egg is inserted into the body. See page 279.

50. *What else needs to be determined before a tubal reversal is considered?*

Your doctor should make sure your separated tubes are the only cause of your infertility. He should make sure your husband is fertile by performing a semen analysis and post-coital test. Surgery should be preceded by a laparoscopy exam to see how much of the tube remains.

51. *How is a laparoscopy exam performed for tubal-reversal surgery?*

It can be done either as a one-stage or two-stage procedure. In a one-stage procedure, a laparoscopy exam is done to determine how much tube is left, then the tubal-reversal surgery is carried out at that time if the doctor feels there is enough tube left to give a good chance of success.

A two-stage procedure involves doing a laparoscopy, evaluating the tubes and discussing the results with you. The tubal reversal is scheduled for another time.

52. *What do the results of surgery depend upon?*

Studies have shown that if you have 5cm (about 2 inches) of tube remaining after tubes are reconnected, the chance for a successful pregnancy is good. If you have less than 3cm of tube present, the outlook is poor. Between 3 and 5cm, the results are only fair. The more tube left, the better the results.

53. *What if I am not a candidate for tubal-reversal surgery?*

If you've had your fimbria or tube removed or there was not enough tube left to reconnect, you may be a candidate for in-vitro fertilization.

54. *How successful are tubal-reversal procedures?*

A doctor experienced in microsurgery can give you an idea of what your chances of success would be. The success rate is about 70 to 80% if surgery is done by an experienced microsurgeon and there is at least 2 inches of tube after reconnection. Before microsurgery, the best success rate was about 50%.

55. *How soon after tubal-reversal surgery should I try to become pregnant?*

It's usually best to try for pregnancy as soon as possible after you recover from surgery and are able to resume sexual intercourse.

56. *Is tubal-reversal surgery expensive?*

Yes, it is. The total cost varies from $5,000 to $10,000 for the surgeon and hospital bills. It is elective surgery, so medical insurance probably will not cover the expense. The use of the operating microscope and the necessity for longer time in the operating room also raise the cost.

57. *Is it better to have a tubal reversal or try in-vitro fertilization?*

If you are a candidate for reversal surgery, it is less expensive and more successful to have reversal surgery than in-vitro fertilization.

58. *What is a vasectomy?*

It is a surgical procedure performed on a man. The vas deferens are cut and separated for permanent sterilization. The surgery keeps sperm from getting into the seminal fluid.

59. *Does a man still ejaculate after having a vasectomy?*

Yes. Most of the ejaculate comes from the seminal vesicles, prostate gland and Cowper's gland, so the only change is there are no sperm present in the ejaculate.

60. *How long does it take to clear the sperm from the male reproductive system after a vasectomy has been performed?*

It may take from just a few ejaculations to 12 to 15 or more. A man must not consider himself sterile until a semen analysis has been done to make sure no sperm are present.

61. *What if a man changes his mind and wants to have more children?*

As in tubal reversals, vasectomy reversals can be done.

62. *How are vasectomy reversals performed?*

It is much easier to separate the vas deferens than to put them back together. This procedure involves a scrotal incision in the area where the vas was tied off and reconnecting the vas deferens after removing scar tissue.

63. *Can microsurgery be used for vasectomy reversals?*

Microsurgery is used in this procedure with good results.

64. *What do results depend upon?*

Success usually depends on the time interval between the original vasectomy and the reversal procedure. If the procedure was done within the previous 5 years, the success rate can be as high as 90%. If it was done longer than 10 years ago, the success rate is less than 50%.

After a vasectomy is performed, the testicles still produce sperm and fluid. Because there is no outlet for sperm, the sperm tend to back up and cause pressure on the epididymis and seminiferous tubules, resulting in damage to these organs. Sperm mature in the epididymis, so the damage that may have been caused by backed-up sperm may result in sperm that are immature, poorly mobile and incapable of fertilization after the reversal. This accounts for the decrease in the success rate due to the time interval from the original vasectomy.

65. *Can other problems develop?*

A man can develop antibodies against his own sperm from the back-up of sperm after the reversal procedure.

66. *How long does it take for sperm to be normal after a reversal?*

Because of the damage to the epididymis and the time needed for recovery, it usually takes between 6 and 24 months for vasectomy reversals to succeed. The sperm count often returns to normal before motility, so don't give up hope if pregnancy is not achieved in the first several months.

67. *If a man is contemplating a vasectomy, is it possible to save sperm for the future?*

Yes. There are sperm banks in most major cities across the United States where this can be done.

68. *How expensive is it to store sperm?*

It costs between $25 and $50 a year.

69. *Do sperm retain their ability to fertilize after being frozen?*

If frozen properly, most of the sperm retain their ability to fertilize. There may be some loss in motility, but for someone with a normal semen analysis, it is probably insignificant. If a man has a borderline semen analysis, his sperm may not freeze well because sperm are already compromised in their ability to fertilize, and freezing is an added stress to these already borderline functioning sperm.

70. *How is sperm used after semen is frozen?*

It is thawed slowly at room temperature, then used for artificial insemination.

71. *Is there any danger in using frozen sperm?*

Extensive studies using animal and human sperm do not reveal any increase in abnormalities in the offspring. It has been established that using frozen sperm from sperm banks is safe.

72. *If a man's body continues to produce sperm after a vasectomy, can sperm be removed from the testicles and used for artificial insemination even after a vasectomy?*

No, they cannot. Sperm in the testicles, rete testis and epididymis are immature and incapable of fertilization. Sperm must be constantly moving along the pathway of the testicles, rete testis, epididymis and vas deferens to maintain their ability to fertilize an egg.

73. *What is an abortion?*

In medical terms, an abortion is the expulsion from the uterus of the contents of pregnancy. If this occurs naturally, it is called a *miscarriage* or *spontaneous abortion*. In layman's terms, an abortion is an elective termination of a pregnancy. In this section, we discuss possible fertility problems following an elective abortion.

74. *How is an abortion performed?*

An abortion is performed by opening the cervix of the uterus with dilators. A plastic tube, which is connected to a suction or vacuum machine, is inserted into the uterine cavity, and the products of pregnancy are removed with the suction tube. A curette is inserted into the uterus to remove any tissue remaining in the uterine cavity.

75. *Can abortions have an affect on future fertility?*

Most abortions performed today are done under safe, legal conditions, and they carry very little risk to a woman's future fertility. Before legalized abortion, the incidence of complications was much greater and could threaten a woman's fertility and her life.

Abortion is a surgical procedure; as with any surgical procedure, possible complications can occur. These complications include infection, uterine perforation and cervical incompetence.

76. *Is fertility affected by an infection following an abortion?*

There is a small chance of infection. Most infections are easily treated with antibiotics and do not result in permanent damage. An inflammation of the uterine lining, called *endometritis,* may occur. If severe, it may result in Asherman's Syndrome. A more severe infection, called salpingitis (inflammation of the Fallopian tubes), or PID may result in permanent damage to the Fallopian tubes because of scarring and blockage.

77. *How do these infections occur?*

Infections can occur from improper abortion technique or not using sterile instruments. A more common cause of infection is performing an abortion through a cervix that is infected with disease, such as gonorrhea or chlamydia.

Dilating the cervix often "stirs up" bacteria, enabling them to move from the cervix into the uterine cavity where they grow and multiply.

78. *Is there any other way to get an infection?*

An abortion that leaves fragments of placenta behind may result in greater risk of an infection.

79. *What is a uterine perforation?*

This is a situation in which the uterus is perforated with dilators or other instruments. Usually a small perforation heals by itself without treatment and has no effect on future fertility. If the perforation is large or in an area where the uterine arteries and veins enter the uterus, an operation may be needed to control bleeding. Rarely, a hysterectomy is needed if bleeding cannot be controlled by any other method.

80. *I've heard cervical incompetence can affect a woman's fertility because she cannot carry a fetus to term. What is cervical incompetence?*

It is a condition in which the cervix is unable to hold a pregnancy within the uterus.

81. *What happens when the cervix cannot hold a pregnancy?*

A premature delivery may occur between the fifth and eighth months of pregnancy.

82. *What causes cervical incompetence?*

It may be a congenital defect or result from trauma or tears in the cervix from a previous delivery or a forceful dilatation from an abortion.

83. *How common is cervical incompetence?*

It is rare but believed to be more common in women who have had repeated abortions. If abortions are properly done, cervical incompetence is rare.

84. *How is cervical incompetence diagnosed?*

If you have had a previous premature delivery, you should be observed closely during pregnancy and have your cervix checked for premature dilatation. Let your doctor know if you have had a previous abortion so your cervix can be checked for premature dilatation.

85. *What can be done if premature dilatation of the cervix is found?*

The doctor can place a stitch around the cervix to prevent it from opening prematurely. This procedure is called a *cervical cerclage.*

13

How Do
Sexually Transmitted Diseases
Affect Fertility?

Sexually transmitted diseases have become more common, and the problems they create affect more people. A sexually transmitted disease can have an impact on a woman's fertility, as well as a man's. Being knowledgeable about the causes and treatments of these diseases will help you understand the impact they have on fertility.

1. *What is a sexually transmitted disease?*

A sexually transmitted disease is a disease transmitted by sexual intercourse. It is also called an *STD* or *venereal disease.*

2. *What are some sexually transmitted diseases?*

The most common ones include gonorrhea, syphilis, chlamydia, ureaplasma, mycoplasma, herpes, condylomata acuminata (venereal warts), hemophilus (gardnerella) and trichomonas infections.

3. *What are the most common sexually transmitted diseases?*

Gonorrhea and chlamydia are the two most common sexually transmitted disease. They have reached epidemic proportions in many areas. Together they cause 80% of all PIDs.

4. *Can a person have more than one sexually transmitted disease?*

It's not uncommon to have several of these diseases at the same time. This becomes important in prescribing treatment to make sure the primary disease is cured and to cure any other sexually transmitted disease that may be present.

5. *What is gonorrhea?*

Gonorrhea is caused by Neisseria gonorrhea bacteria; the disease can affect the cervix, urethra, rectum and anal canal. Gonorrhea can be transmitted from the genital organs to the throat by oral sex.

6. *What are the symptoms of gonorrhea in a woman?*

A vaginal discharge may be present. If the infection progresses into the uterus and Fallopian tubes, it can cause PID, resulting in abdominal pain and fever. Women may carry the gonorrhea organism in the cervix without symptoms.

7. *What are the symptoms of gonorrhea in a man?*

In the majority of cases, a man has a discharge from the penis. We now realize that men, as well as women, can carry gonorrhea without symptoms.

8. *How does gonorrhea affect a woman?*

Gonorrhea may remain localized in the cervix where it can cause a purulent cervicitis (pus-filled, inflamed cervix), which causes a vaginal discharge. It can also go into the uterus and Fallopian tubes and cause salpingitis (inflammation of the Fallopian tubes) or PID.

Gonorrhea can spread through the entire body by way of the bloodstream and cause a gonococcal infection anywhere in the body. Infection may be found in the joints (causing arthritis), in the skin (causing rashes) or involve the heart lining (causing endocarditis).

9. *How does gonorrhea affect a man?*

It can cause inflammation of the penile urethra, leading to a pus-filled discharge from the penis. Infection can also spread through the bloodstream to affect distant organs, such as joints, skin and heart, as in a woman.

10. *How does gonorrhea affect fertility in a woman?*

If the cervix is involved, infection causes poor cervical mucus, and sperm are unable to swim through the cervical canal. If tubes become infected with gonorrhea, they may become permanently scarred. Adhesions and scarring may interfere with tubal function and may possibly cause blockages in them.

11. *How does gonorrhea affect fertility in a man?*

Gonorrhea can cause a narrowing of the urethra, which may result in difficultly urinating. It can also involve the ductal system and cause blockage in the vas deferens or epididymis. Blockage of the vas deferens is more serious because it keeps sperm from getting into the ejaculate.

12. *What is chlamydia?*

Chlamydia is a bacterial infection caused by chlamydia trachomatis. It is presently the most common sexually transmitted disease and is more common than gonorrhea, herpes and mycoplasma combined.

13. *What are the symptoms of chlamydia in a woman?*

In women, chlamydia may cause a cervicitis similar to gonorrhea, with a vaginal discharge. Many women do not have any symptoms at all. Similar to gonorrhea, chlamydia can cause an infection of the uterine lining and PID. Chlamydia also causes formation of scar tissue around the tubes and ovaries. Silent PID is becoming more common with chlamydial infections.

14. *What are the symptoms of chlamydia in a man?*

The main symptoms include burning during urination and a milky discharge from the penis.

15. *How common is chlamydia?*

It is very common. As many as 20 to 40% of *all* sexually active women have been exposed to chlamydia. Fifteen to 25% of all women have chlamydia and do not know it.

16. *Why is there such a high rate?*

The majority of women with chlamydia have few symptoms or no symptoms at all. The incubation period is about 10 days; a persistent carrier state (a person who chronically carries a disease without knowing it) can exist. Many women do not know they have chlamydia unless their partner develops symptoms.

17. *How can chlamydia affect fertility in a woman or a man?*

In a woman, it can cause poor cervical mucus and possible tubal damage. In a man, it can cause a blockage of the vas deferens and epididymis, which results in few, if any, sperm in the semen.

18. *Does the method of birth control affect chlamydia?*

Women who use oral contraceptives have a higher incidence of chlamydial infections. There are two reasons for this.

1. Barrier methods of birth control, such as condoms or a diaphragm, provide protection from transmitting or contracting sexually transmitted diseases.

2. Women who are on the pill are more likely to develop a cervical eversion.

19. *What is a cervical eversion?*

Cervical eversion is a condition in which mucus-producing cells that normally line the endocervix extend onto the exocervix. This allows bacteria to get into the cervical glands more easily to cause cervicitis. The presence of a cervical eversion is why some women on birth-control pills have increased discharge, even without an infection.

20. *Can a person have gonorrhea and chlamydia without knowing it?*

Yes. Men *and* women can have gonorrhea or chlamydia for a long time without any symptoms. Several years ago, it was believed if men had these diseases, they would have a discharge from the penis. We now know men and women can be free of symptoms and still carry sexually transmitted diseases.

21. *How are gonorrhea and chlamydia treated?*

Antibiotics, such as penicillin, erythromycin and tetracycline, are usually effective against gonorrhea. Chlamydia is usually treated with tetracycline. Your doctor knows the best medication for you.

Because there is such a high incidence of these diseases existing together, it's important to prescribe antibiotics that work against *both* organisms. This is especially true when gonorrhea is found because treating gonorrhea with penicillin is fine for the gonorrhea, but it does not work against chlamydia. Many doctors follow penicillin treatment of gonorrhea with an oral course of tetracycline to treat chlamydia if it should be present.

22. *Should both partners be treated for a sexually transmitted disease?*

Yes. If you have had recent sexual contact with someone with a sexually transmitted disease, you should be treated as if you have the disease. It is advisable to treat both partners, even though the disease is only found in one of them.

23. *How are serious problems, such as tubal blockage and adhesions, treated in a woman?*

If you have tubal blockage or adhesions, surgery may be necessary for pregnancy to occur. If tubes are permanently damaged, you may be a candidate for in-vitro fertilization.

24. *How is ductal blockage treated in a man?*

If ductal blockage is present in a man, microsurgery may be necessary to bypass the blockage. If numerous blockages are present, there may be no treatment.

25. *What is syphilis?*

Syphilis is a sexually transmitted disease that begins as a non-tender sore called a *chancre*. A chancre is the primary lesion of syphilis that develops at the site of entrance of the infection. It appears as a small papule that erodes into an ulcer that is covered with a yellowish discharge. This sore is usually located on the genitals. In about 5% of the cases, a chancre can be found on the lips, breast or mouth—it may be the only sore a person gets.

If this stage goes undetected, syphilis can develop into a widespread skin rash or large, wartlike growths on the genitals called *condylomata lata* (not to be confused with venereal warts or condylomata accuminata).

If the disease is left untreated for more than a year, it can involve any organ in the body. Syphilis can involve the brain and spinal cord 10 to 20 years after exposure, which may affect a person's mental state and cause difficulty in walking. Involvement of the heart and heart valves can occur 20 to 30 years after first being exposed.

26. *Does syphilis affect fertility?*

Early syphilis does not affect a woman's ability to become pregnant, but it can affect the developing baby if left untreated during pregnancy.

27. *How is syphilis treated?*

The primary treatment of syphilis is penicillin.

28. *What if a person is allergic to penicillin?*

If a person is allergic to penicillin, erythromycin or tetracycline can be used. The dosage and type of antibiotic depends on the stage of the disease when it is diagnosed.

29. *What is genital herpes?*

Genital herpes is a viral disease that can result in sores anywhere on the genital organs. It affects men and women. It usually begins 3 to 6 days after exposure and results in small, fluid-filled sores similar to early chicken pox. The skin over these sores breaks down and becomes very painful. Other symptoms, such as chills, fever and tender lymph glands, may also occur. After 7 to 14 days, sores heal without scarring.

30. *Are there other types of herpes infections?*

There are many different types of herpes viruses, which are similar to the chicken-pox virus. They cause many illnesses, such as shingles (herpes zoster), which is a disease that can cause severe pain and a rash. A cold sore and cankers in the mouth are also caused by a herpes virus.

31. *Can oral herpes be transmitted to the genital area?*

Yes. If a person has oral sex with an open cold sore or active canker, it is possible to transmit the oral form of herpes to the genital area. The oral form of herpes is believed to be caused by the Type-1 herpes virus; the genital form is caused by the Type-2 herpes virus.

It is becoming common for the Type-1 virus to cause genital herpes and Type-2 virus to cause oral herpes. It doesn't make any difference which type of herpes you get in the genital area. Classifying the type of herpes is a research tool to differentiate the viruses. Treatment, cure rate and recurrence rate is the same for both.

32. *How is herpes diagnosed?*

It is usually diagnosed by the presence of open, active sores, preceded by a 1-to-2 day episode of burning or itching in the area involved. A culture can be done to confirm the diagnosis. An initial bout of herpes may be so small it can go undetected. The only way a person eventually knows he or she has the disease is if there is a recurrence without a history of recent sexual contact.

33. *Do herpes recur?*

Once you get herpes, the virus often remains in the nerve roots where the infection first occurred. Recurrences may occur without any new exposure to the virus. Although recurrences are much less painful than the first attack, and are shorter in duration, they are annoying to the person infected. Herpes can be contagious in the active phase and the presymptom stage of the disease 3 to 6 days after exposure. Symptoms may be so mild you may not realize you have herpes and pass it on through sexual contact. Everyone who gets herpes does *not* get recurrences—the initial bout may be all you ever get. At this time, we don't know what makes herpes recur.

34. *Do certain conditions bring on recurrences?*

It appears stress may cause recurrences. Women also appear to break out with periodic episodes during the same part of their menstrual cycle. This may occur monthly or only a few times a year.

35. *What is the treatment for herpes?*

There is no treatment to prevent recurrences of the disease. Acyclovir, available in cream and pill form, can be taken at the onset of symptoms; it may shorten the duration and reduce the severity of herpes. Oral acyclovir can also be taken daily to help prevent recurrence, but it cannot be taken during pregnancy.

36. *Does herpes affect fertility?*

Herpes does not appear to affect fertility. If a person has herpes, he or she might be too sore to have intercourse if active sores are present.

The real danger with herpes is in a pregnant woman; a baby should *not* be delivered through the birth canal if an active herpes sore is present. A newborn infected with herpes can become seriously ill, with a death rate of 25 to 50%. Mental retardation and developmental problems may also occur.

If an active herpes sore is present at the time a woman goes into labor or is at term, a Cesarean section is the preferred method of delivery.

37. *What are venereal warts?*

Venereal warts (condylomata accuminata) are small warts caused by a virus called *papillovirus*. They can occur anywhere on the penis or urethra in a man and anywhere on the external female genitalia, vagina and cervix in a woman. Warts can also occur in the anal canal in both sexes.

38. *How does someone get venereal warts?*

Warts are contracted from contact with the papillo-virus, usually by sexual intercourse.

39. *Do venereal warts interfere with fertility?*

They don't interfere with conception, but in women warts may increase in size during pregnancy because their growth is stimulated by hormones of pregnancy. Warts may obstruct the birth canal, and a Cesarean section may be necessary. A baby born to a mother with active warts may be more likely to get polyps on his larynx.

40. *How are warts treated?*

Podophyllin or various acids, such as bichloracetic, trichloracetic acid and salicylic acid, have been used with good results. In widespread or resistant cases, carbon-dioxide laser may be used. Warts may also be cauterized, frozen or surgically removed.

41. *What are mycoplasma and ureaplasma infections?*

Mycoplasma hominis and ureaplasma urealyticum are bacterialike organisms that have recently been found to be a common cause of cervicitis and PID in women and urethritis in men. The ureaplasma organism was previously called T-mycoplasma (T for tiny). Other types of mycoplasma are also present but rarely infect humans; they commonly infect animals.

42. *How can mycoplasma and ureaplasma infections affect a woman's fertility?*

Mycoplasma and ureaplamsa infections have been implicated in cervicitis, PID, miscarriages and infertility. They cause poor cervical mucus and tubal damage.

43. *Can mycoplasma and ureaplasma infections affect a man's fertility?*

Yes. They have been shown to cause non-specific urethritis and prostatitis. If the prostate gland is affected, infections can affect sperm motility and cause agglutination of sperm.

44. *How can mycoplasma and ureaplasma infections be diagnosed?*

Cultures for mycoplasma and ureaplasma are done for both partners. This is often part of an infertility investigation, even if symptoms do not exist. The organism may be present in the urethra, prostate or cervix without symptoms. This may be a factor in causing infertility.

45. *How are mycoplasma and ureaplasma infections treated?*

Tetracycline is the treatment of choice. Both partners are usually treated for 7 to 14 days, even if the organism is found in only one. Some researchers have treated couples who have unexplained infertility with tetracycline to see if this will improve fertility, even though cultures are negative. It is unknown at this time if this type of treatment has increased the pregnancy rate.

46. *What is a hemophilus infection?*

It is a vaginal infection caused by the organism hemophilus vaginalis; it is also called *gardnerella vaginalis* or *non-specific vaginitis.*

47. *What are the symptoms of hemophilus infections?*

In a woman, symptoms may include a light-green vaginal discharge associated with vaginal itching and a fishy odor. In a man, hemophilus is believed to be one of the organisms responsible for non-specific urethritis and prostatitis.

48. *How is a hemophilus infection diagnosed?*

Your doctor examines your vaginal discharge for clue cells. *Clue cells* are vaginal epitheliial cells covered with tiny bacteria. If a hemophilus infection is present, the clue cells are the predominant cells seen when a smear is examined under the microscope.

49. *How is hemophilus vaginitis treated?*

Tetracycline or metronidazole are the best treatments. A sulfa-based vaginal cream may be used, but it isn't as effective.

50. *Are both partners treated?*

It is best to treat both partners even if hemophilus is found in only one.

51. *Does hemophilus interfere with fertility?*

A mild hemophilus infection probably does not. If severe, an infection can alter the acidity of the vagina and change the quality of the cervical mucus. This makes it difficult for sperm to survive. In a man, hemophilus may cause a decrease in sperm motility and agglutination of sperm.

52. *What is a trichomonas infection?*

It is a vaginal infection caused by a single-celled organism called *trichomonas vaginalis*. It is chiefly transmitted by sexual intercourse, although occasional infestation from spas or hot tubs or contamination by bath articles or toilet seats has been reported.

53. *What are the symptoms of a trichomonas infection?*

In a woman, it can cause severe inflammation in the vagina and severe itching in the external genital area. In a man, it can cause burning during urination. Men and women can have a trichomonas infection without symptoms.

54. *How is a trichomonas infection diagnosed?*

It is diagnosed by examining vaginal secretions for the trichomonas organism.

55. *How is a trichomonas infection treated?*

It is treated with the antibiotic metronidazole, which is one antibiotic also used for hemophilus infections.

56. *Do trichomonas infections affect fertility?*

Possibly. If you have a trichomonas infection, it may cause local irritation and make intercourse difficult and uncomfortable. It can also change the acidity of the vagina, cause poor cervical mucus and affect sperm survival.

57. *Can sexually transmitted diseases be prevented?*

The use of condoms has been shown to be the best method of preventing sexually transmitted diseases. A condom protects a man from getting a disease from a woman, and a woman is protected from getting a sexually transmitted disease from a man. As soon as a person has more than one sexual partner, the chances of contracting a sexually transmitted disease rises sharply. A diaphragm also provides some protection but not as much as a condom.

58. *Are there general symptoms that would alert me to a sexually transmitted disease?*

A woman should suspect she may have a sexually transmitted disease if she has an unusual, odorous, vaginal discharge or any sores present on the genitals. A man may have STD if he has sores, burning with urination or a discharge from the penis.

59. *What does the future hold for prevention of sexually transmitted diseases?*

Education about various diseases and how they are transmitted probably holds the most hope for prevention. By being more open and honest with your sexual partner about STD and taking precautions, such as using a condom, will do the most in preventing the spread of disease.

Vaccines against herpes and other STDs are in the developmental stages. They should help control the spread of these diseases in the future, once vaccines are perfected.

60. *What is a yeast infection?*

A yeast or monilia infection is the most common vaginal infection in a woman. It is not considered a sexually transmitted disease but can be confused with one because of its symptoms. A yeast infection can occur in any woman under the right circumstances. Every woman has potential yeast organisms in her vagina; some women are more susceptible to yeast infections than others.

61. *What are the symptoms of a yeast infection?*

A yeast infection causes a white, cottage-cheese type vaginal discharge, with extreme vaginal and vulvar burning and itching.

62. *How is a yeast infection diagnosed?*

It is diagnosed the same way as other vaginal infections—vaginal discharge must be examined.

63. *Under what conditions are yeast infections more common?*

Yeast infections are more common in women who:
- Take antibiotics.
- Have diabetes.
- Are pregnant.
- Take birth-control pills.

64. *What is the treatment of yeast infections?*

The infection is treated locally with a vaginal cream or suppository that kills the yeast organism rather than an antibiotic taken orally.

65. *Why do women who take antibiotics become susceptible to yeast infections?*

Antibiotics kill the intended organism and kill the bacteria normally present in the vagina. This enables yeast organisms to monopolize the vagina and grow and multiply, which often results in an infection. When other vaginal infections are treated with antibiotics, it may be wise to use a vaginal yeast medication to prevent a yeast infection from developing.

66. *Do yeast infections affect fertility?*

Mild infections probably do not. Severe infections can make intercourse difficult and may interfere with sperm survival and the quality of the mucus.

67. *Do men get yeast infections?*

Men may get external penile skin irritations if they have intercourse with a woman who has a yeast infection. Athlete's foot and jock itch are common yeast infections men are prone to.

68. *How are men treated for yeast infections?*

A man can be treated with the same cream a woman uses for her infection.

69. *Do yeast infections affect a man's fertility?*

No, yeast infections do not affect a man's fertility.

14
What Medical Advances Have Been Made in Infertility?

As in most areas of medicine, infertility research is making slow but steady progress. Since 1978, when the first test-tube baby was born, we have seen many new developments and "spin-offs" from that procedure.

What is considered experimental and "for research" today will hopefully be common practice in the near future and give hope to many infertile couples.

1. *What is in-vitro fertilization?*

In-vitro fertilization is the process in which a pregnancy is achieved by combining sperm and the egg outside a woman's body in a laboratory dish. The dish contains special nutrients so the egg can develop and make its first few cell divisions. The fertilized egg is implanted into the uterine lining of the mother-to-be.

In-vitro means in a test tube or in a glass. Another common name for this procedure is *test-tube baby*.

2. *How is in-vitro fertilization performed?*

A laparoscopy examination is performed on you at ovulation to obtain several ripe eggs. Prior to laparoscopy, you may have been given ovarian-stimulating drugs, such as Pergonal or Clomid, to mature several eggs at the same time.

Sperm is obtained from your husband and may be treated with one of the sperm-washing techniques to improve the sperm's chances for fertilizing the eggs.

Eggs and sperm are mixed in a petri dish, then placed in an incubator for 2 to 3 days where the fertilized eggs divide and develop into an 8-to-16 cell embryo called a *morula.* The morula is then inserted into the uterus by placing a small tube through the vagina and cervix and injecting the morula into the uterine cavity. Hopefully the morula will implant on the uterine lining.

Often several developing embryos are placed in the uterus for a better chance of at least one fertilized egg implanting and developing.

3. *Who are candidates for in-vitro fertilization?*

It was originally intended for women with irreparably blocked Fallopian tubes. Today, in-vitro fertilization is being used for other causes of infertility, such as in immunologic and unexplained infertility, and male-factor infertility (low sperm count, poor sperm motility) with improving results.

4. *If I have blocked Fallopian tubes, do I have a better chance of conceiving if I have reversal surgery or in-vitro fertilization?*

It depends on the degree of blockage and the severity of adhesions. If you had tubal sterilization, reversal surgery usually gives a greater chance of success. If there is severe, irreparable blockage, you are probably a candidate for in-vitro fertilization.

5. *Can sperm be used from someone other than the husband?*

Yes, donor sperm can be used. This is similar to artificial insemination using donor sperm.

6. *Where is in-vitro fertilization performed?*

There are over 175 clinics in the United States where in-vitro fertilization is performed. Your doctor will know the closest clinic and the success rate of that clinic.

7. *How expensive is the procedure?*

It costs $5,000 to $6,000 for *one attempt* at in-vitro fertilization.

8. *Why is it so expensive?*

In-vitro fertilization is a very technical procedure requiring laparoscopy for egg retrieval, daily serum-estrogen levels and several ultrasound examinations each month to see the developing eggs.

Infertility specialists and professionals who are in charge of sperm and ovum specimens are also involved in the procedure.

9. *What is the success rate of the procedure?*

The overall success rate of any cycle is only about 10 to 12%. There is only 1 chance in 10 of becoming pregnant from a single attempt at in-vitro fertilization.

10. *Do some clinics have a higher success rate than others?*

More-experienced clinics usually have a higher success rate. As more is learned about the procedure, the success rate will improve. One recent report showed a 30 to 35% success rate in selected patients, which is a marked improvement over earlier reports.

11. *How many babies have been born by this method?*

Since Louise Brown (the first test-tube baby) was born in England in 1978, there have been over 1,000 babies born worldwide by this procedure. In the United States, the first clinic was established at the Eastern Virginia Medical School in Norfolk, Virginia; it has had the greatest success—150 babies, with 20 sets of twins and 2 sets of triplets.

12. *What is meant by in-vivo fertilization?*

In-vivo means within the body, in contrast to *in-vitro*, which means outside the body. In-vivo fertilization involves removing an egg by laparoscopy, mixing it with washed sperm from the husband and immediately placing the washed sperm and egg back into the Fallopian tube. This is all done in the same laparoscopy procedure.

Fertilization takes place in the Fallopian tube and goes on to implant in the uterine cavity. This method of in-vivo fertilization is called **GIFT**—gamete intra-Fallopian transfer.

13. *Who are candidates for the GIFT procedure?*

GIFT is presently being used in some fertility clinics for couples with unexplained infertility, male-factor infertility and in some cases of endometriosis. You must have one functioning tube to be a candidate for this procedure.

14. *Are there other methods of in-vivo fertilization?*

There are three methods that have been used for in-vivo fertilization.

1. Intratubal insemination is placing washed sperm directly into the Fallopian tube during a laparoscopy after spontaneous or stimulated ovulation. The egg is ovulated normally into the Fallopian tube where previously placed sperm from the husband await the egg's arrival. This procedure is unlike in-vitro fertilization but similar to GIFT; it requires at least one functioning Fallopian tube.

2. Treated, washed sperm from the husband can be placed directly into the Fallopian tube with a hysteroscope. If this is successful, there is no need for laparoscopy. This procedure can be performed in a doctor's office.

3. During laparoscopy, eggs are transferred from the

ovary to the Fallopian tube where they may be fertilized by waiting sperm.

Despite reported cases of pregnancy using all of these techniques, in-vivo fertilization is considered experimental at this time but may hold considerable hope for the future.

15. *What is a donor-embryo transfer?*

It is a technique used for women who cannot produce eggs but can carry a fetus. A woman who is willing to donate her eggs is found; she must be at the same part of the menstrual cycle as the woman who will receive the embryo. This may require using Clomid in both women.

The donor is artificially inseminated with the husband's sperm. Five to 7 days after insemination, when the fertilized egg first enters the uterine cavity, a special catheter is placed into the uterine cavity of the donor to retrieve the fertilized egg. The fertilized egg is then placed into the wife's uterus using the same technique as embryo transfer in in-vitro fertilization.

16. *Genetically, who does the baby resemble?*

The egg comes from the donor female, so it will have genes from the donor, not the wife. The sperm is from the husband, so it will have his genes.

17. *What is a surrogate mother?*

Surrogate means *substitute*. A surrogate mother is a woman who carries a pregnancy to term for another couple.

18. *How does the surrogate mother become pregnant?*

A surrogate mother can be artificially inseminated with a husband's sperm, carry the pregnancy to term, then give the baby back to the couple.

19. *Genetically, who does the baby resemble?*

The genetic makeup of the infant would be that of the husband and surrogate mother.

20. *Is there another way for a surrogate mother to become pregnant?*

A woman who had her uterus removed donates an egg (by laparoscopy), and the egg is fertilized with her husband's sperm. The fertilized egg is then placed into the uterus of a surrogate mother. The surrogate mother has the baby then gives it back to the couple.

21. *Genetically, who will this baby resemble?*

This child would have the genetic makeup of the couple. The surrogate mother is a carrier of the baby and does not contribute to his genetic makeup.

22. *Why would a woman act as an egg donor or surrogate mother?*

The incentive is usually money. These women are paid well, usually thousands of dollars, to be a surrogate mother. In addition, the medical expenses for the pregnancy are paid for by the couple.

23. *Are there potential problems with surrogate-mother pregnancies?*

There is a possibility an agreement between the parents and surrogate mother will not be honored. There are cases in which the surrogate mother did not give the baby to the parents as promised, despite legal contracts signed beforehand.

24. *What is a frozen embryo?*

A frozen embryo is a frozen fertilized egg; it is frozen after fertilization and the first few cell divisions and saved for future use.

25. *How are frozen embryos obtained?*

They are obtained in a manner similar to the procedure for in-vitro fertilization. Eggs are obtained by laparoscopy, mixed with sperm so fertilization can occur and frozen for later use.

26. *How are frozen embryos used?*

They can be used by a couple to have their own child, after one or both of them have become sterile. They can be also used in in-vitro fertilization so the woman does not have to undergo a laparoscopy each month to retrieve new eggs. She would only have to undergo an embryo transfer in subsequent months to attempt pregnancy.

The use of frozen embryos can greatly reduce costs of in-vitro fertilization because laparoscopy would not have to be done each month. Several eggs can be obtained during one laparoscopy exam, then used during the next several cycles.

The issue of frozen embryos raises many moral and ethical questions, such as to whom these frozen embryos would belong if the original parents are no longer living. These and other issues must be addressed if frozen embryos are to be used in the future.

15
How Can We Cope with the Emotional Effects of Infertility?

In addition to the physical impact of infertility—no pregnancy—there is also an emotional impact. Every couple we have interviewed expressed the same feelings, fears and frustrations. They said they felt as if they were on an emotional merry-go-round; the longer their infertility went on, the harder it was to cope.

It is often embarrassing to admit you have a problem, and it's difficult to admit your physical problem affects you emotionally. It's hard for other people to understand infertility. We hope you can find some answers in this section about coping with well-meaning family and friends.

Your emotional turmoil may affect your relationship with your spouse, your family and your friends. We know your feelings and emotions are real, and they must be dealt with. You aren't alone!

Below is a checklist of feelings. How many of them have you experienced?

Do you find yourself:

• Asking your husband's forgiveness, saying "I'm getting my period."?

• Saying you missed the right day of the month and had intercourse the wrong day?

• Experiencing irritability and fatigue while making love during midcycle?

• Not in the mood to make love?

• Losing the stamina to stand up to the stress and pain of infertility?

• So preoccupied with infertility that everything else in your life suffers?

• Feeling that nothing in your life is fulfilling?

• Feeling you let each other down?

• Feeling you want to take a break from trying to conceive but don't know how to tell your spouse?

• Having feelings of shock, disbelief, sadness and disappointment each month?

• Feeling totally out of control with the situation?

• Feeling discriminated against because you don't have children?

• Feeling infertility is never-ending?

You're experiencing normal feelings and frustrations. Face them and talk about them. You're feeling what others have felt—let them help you.

1. *I feel happy and sad when I hear someone else is pregnant. Why?*

You're being honest about your feelings. It's normal to feel happiness and resentment at the same time. You're happy for them but depressed for yourself.

2. *Why do my feelings fluctuate?*

It's not uncommon to become frustrated, jealous, impatient, angry and depressed—all at the same time. You're normal, and you're expressing your emotions.

3. *Why is it so hard to talk about my feelings?*

It takes courage to talk about what you're feeling, and it takes longer for some people to gather their courage. Once you can talk about your feelings, you may find things are not so bad, or that they could be a lot worse.

4. *I feel as if I'm being punished for past mistakes. Am I?*

It's easier to have a reason for why something isn't happening, but it's nonsense. Don't blame yourself for past mistakes.

5. *We are both experiencing feelings of guilt and pressure. Is this normal?*

If either of you are feeling guilty or feeling pressured, sit down and talk. You need to be mutually supportive of each other. Discuss how you feel.

6. *I feel as if we're unable to help each other. What can we do?*

It's time to seek outside help.

7. *What kind of help should we look for?*

You can seek professional counseling, join a support group or talk with people who have experienced infertility. Many professional counselors today are specializing in infertile-couple counseling.

8. *Where do we go to find help?*

Your doctor may be able to direct you to a counselor. Family and friends may know of other couples who have experienced infertility. There is a support group in most states called *Resolve.*

9. *How do we get in touch with Resolve in our area?*

Look in the telephone directory, or write to:
Resolve, Inc.
P.O. Box 474
Belmont, MA 02178

10. *Can infertility problems be sexual?*

Pregnancy can be avoided by purposely avoiding intercourse.

11. *Is it uncommon to have infrequent sexual relations?*

No. Infrequent sexual relations can be caused by health, fatigue, work schedules and other situations.

12. *Can anxieties lead to physical problems so intercourse is impossible?*

Yes. A woman can develop a spasm of the vaginal muscles (vaginismus), making it impossible for a man to enter sexually. A man may not be able to have an erection (impotence) because of anxieties; this makes intercourse impossible.

13. *Are these common conditions?*

Vaginismus occurs occasionally at the start of a marriage. Impotence can happen at any time.

14. *I feel like I'm a robot when we make love. Is this normal?*

This is a common feeling because you are having sex to reach a goal, not only for the sake of making love.

15. *Do other couples feel their sex life is no longer private?*

Yes, because when you experience infertility, sex is often discussed with your doctor.

16. *I find it hard to discuss my sex life with my doctor. What can I do?*

This is a common problem. If you're uncomfortable discussing it with your doctor, tell him how you feel. If your doctor isn't sensitive to your feelings, you might have to find another doctor.

17. *Do other couples find their sex life is no longer exciting?*

This is probably the most common complaint because you feel as if you are having "sex on demand."

18. *What can we do to make our sex life more exciting?*

Create some new techniques to make sex more exciting. Often different intercourse positions and longer foreplay will give both of you renewed sexual pleasure.

19. *I'm so bored nothing seems to help. Is there something we can do?*

You might have to take a break from trying to conceive.

20. *We both feel bored and sexually inadequate. Do others feel the same way?*

Infertility doesn't mean you are sexually inadequate. It only means you aren't conceiving.

21. *What effects can infertility have on our marriage?*

It can bind you closer together. It can also cause negative effects on a marriage, such as anxiety, pain, financial stress and sexual hostility.

22. *We look at ourselves as failures. Are we?*

Some people feel that way, but that's unfair to you. Each month you go through the agonizing waiting, hoping your period doesn't come. If it does, you feel as though you failed in some way. But you must remember you are *not* failures.

23. *Can infertility lead to stress and tension in a marriage?*

Yes, especially after many months of trying to conceive without success.

24. *Do men tend to hide their reactions?*

Men take infertility seriously, but they often find it difficult to express their feelings.

25. *Is it usually easier for a woman to discuss her infertility?*

Yes. This may be because women seem to have an easier time expressing their feelings.

26. *Our failure to conceive makes me feel like we're "targets of pressure." How do we deal with this?*

Unfortunately, you may get pressure from people who don't understand your infertility problem. Talk to them, and try to make them understand what you are feeling as you deal with your situation.

27. *Should we postpone future plans and dwell only on pregnancy?*

Don't postpone any future plans. If you do become pregnant, plans can be postponed or changed.

28. *Is it possible for us to create our infertility by dwelling on it too much?*

There is no evidence to support this, although severe stress may interplay with your menstrual cycle or ovulation pattern.

29. *Why do well-meaning friends and family pressure us, even if we choose not to discuss our infertility?*

They probably don't realize it bothers you, and they are curious.

30. *Why do family and friends keep offering well-meaning advice when we haven't asked for it?*

It's only natural for friends and family to offer advice. Tell them you need their support not their advice.

31. *If we can't cope with other people's joys, how should we deal with family and friends?*

Be with people, but do something positive for yourself. Then you have a joy to share with them.

32. *Why do people ask inappropriate questions?*

Often they don't know what else to say.

33. *Should we attend family events if we are uncomfortable?*

Family events can become painful, especially if children attend. If family gatherings become too painful, don't go. Hopefully, your hosts will understand.

34. *What if we must attend them?*

You and your husband are a family unit, so try to remember that.

35. *Why do we feel we can't make it through another holiday without a child?*

Holidays aren't perfect for everyone. You might be experiencing infertility, but someone else may be far from home. Try to enjoy the holidays; don't rob yourself of the holiday spirit.

36. *Why is it so hard for people to understand our loneliness?*

Because people do not understand infertility.

37. *What can we do to make people understand how we feel?*

Begin to share your feelings with family and friends. They will have a better understanding of what you are experiencing.

38. *Why do people say, "Having a baby is so easy!"?*

This statement comes from people who have never had children or tried to have children, or from those who didn't have a problem conceiving.

39. *Why do I get depressed every time I see a pregnant woman?*

Because you're jealous; being jealous is a normal reaction.

40. *Why is it that all of our friends seem so fertile?*

It might seem that way to you, but you really don't know how long it took them to become pregnant and what problems they experienced.

41. *Why do friends and family always say infertility is my fault?*

That's false judgment. Ignore it, or explain to them infertility is a combined problem.

42. *When should we stop trying to have a baby and begin to consider alternatives?*

If you have experienced 3 or more years of infertility, after a full evaluation and treatment, you have a poor outlook. The time to consider alternatives depends on you and your husband. Read the following section for further information.

16

How Do We Adopt a Child?

Adoption is an alternative you might consider if you are unable to conceive. Adoption isn't for everyone, but it is the solution for many childless couples around the world.

1. *When should adoption be considered?*

It varies for each couple—it depends on your age and how eager you are to adopt. It may take a few years to adopt a child from the time the adoption procedure is initiated. It may be best to begin as soon as an infertility evaluation indicates your chances for conception are marginal.

2. *Is it easier to become pregnant after a child is adopted?*

That's an old wives' tale. Some people believe once a child is adopted, the stress of becoming pregnant is relieved and a couple can conceive. Infertile couples should never put their hopes on becoming pregnant by adopting a child. The spontaneous cure rate for infertile couples is the same, whether they adopt or not.

3. *Are children available to be adopted?*

Adopting a caucasian infant has become more difficult since 1970. There are many reasons for this—more accessible birth control, the change in the abortion laws and many single women (about 80%) keep their babies.

4. *How long do we have to wait for a baby?*

The wait for a young, healthy infant varies from 6 months to 5 years. The average wait is 18 to 24 months. The length of time it takes to get a baby depends on where you live, the agency you choose, how large an area the agency encompasses and the type of child you adopt.

5. *Are certain children easier to adopt than others?*

Healthy, young infants and preschool children are in very short supply. Older children with medical or emotional handicaps are usually available for adoption in most states. Some of these children may be mentally retarded or have learning disorders.

In the last several years, adopting young, healthy infants from foreign countries has become popular. These children are more available than children from the United States.

6. *From which foreign countries are children being adopted?*

The largest number of readily available children are from Korea, Colombia, India, Thailand, El Salvador and Sri Lanka.

7. *How do I find an adoption agency?*

The names of adoption agencies can be obtained from your state or county Department of Public Welfare, from the Yellow Pages of the phone book listed under *Adoption* or *Social Service Organizations* or from couples who have previously adopted a child.

8. *What types of adoption agencies are there?*

An adoption agency can be public or private, non-profit or for-profit, and licensed or unlicensed. An example of a public, non-profit agency is a county or state government agency. Most large county public welfare offices have an adoption division.

There are also licensed, private adoption agencies in large cities. Many private religious and non-religious agencies are in operation.

9. *What are some licensed, private, religious agencies?*

Catholic Social Services, Lutheran Social Services and Jewish Family Services are a few examples. Most religious agencies handle adoptions of their respective religion, other religions and foreign adoptions.

10. *What are examples of licensed, private, non-religious agencies?*

Children's Home Society and Crossroads are private, non-religious agencies. The names of these agencies vary from city to city. Most large cities have several licensed, private (both non-profit and for-profit) agencies that can give more information on adoption. Some agencies may specialize in foreign adoptions from certain countries.

11. *What is a private adoption?*

In this situation, an attorney or physician acts as an intermediary between a birth mother and an adopting couple. This type of adoption is not legal in every state. An attorney or licensed adoption agency can provide information if this type of adoption is legal in your state.

12. *What are black-market adoptions?*

A black-market adoption is the illegal sale of a baby for profit. This is mentioned *only* to discourage it! It's usually very expensive ($25,000 and up) and carries the risk of possible blackmail or reclamation of the baby by the birth mother or the people who arranged the adoption.

13. *What can we expect when we contact an adoption agency?*

Procedures vary greatly, depending on the agency. You may be invited to an information session that covers topics of interest to an adopting couple, such as children available, the waiting period, requirements for adoptive parents and the procedure the agency requires to adopt a child.

14. *What follows the initial meeting?*

Procedures vary from agency to agency, so it's difficult to generalize. Most agencies require a home study and interviews with the adoptive couple, either individually or jointly.

The agency is the advocate for the adopted child, so it's interested in your lifestyle, your financial security, your health, your reasons for adopting and your attitudes toward raising children.

15. *What is a home study?*

In a home study, a social worker from the adoption agency comes to your home for a series of interviews. It is a shared process between the adoption agency and the adoptive parents. Some social workers drop in unannounced, but they are evaluating you, not your housekeeping abilities, so don't be upset if this happens.

16. *Is it harder to adopt if we already have children?*

No, this is usually not a factor. Some birth parents prefer homes that already have children.

17. *If we have children, will they be interviewed by the agency?*

The agency usually wants to interview your children.

18. *Should we apply to more than one agency?*

Although it may be a good idea to initially contact several agencies for information, it's best to select one agency to work with. Most agencies prefer this. It's expensive and time consuming for the agency to carry out the investigative work in anticipation of placement, then discover you have arranged for a child through another source.

19. *What happens after the interviews and home studies?*

The agency evaluates your application and the recommendations from the social worker who performed the interviews for a final decision as to whether they will accept you as an adoptive couple. If you're accepted, you are put on a waiting list for a baby.

20. *What happens when a child is found?*

The agency calls and tells you they have a child for you to consider for adoption.

21. *Are we given information about the child?*

Yes, you are given as complete information as is possible regarding the child's birth record, illnesses and other significant history.

22. *Do we have to accept the child?*

No, you do not.

23. *If we accept the child, how long do we have to wait before the child is legally ours?*

In most states, the waiting period is 6 months, but it can be from 2 weeks to 1 year, sometimes longer. The procedure varies greatly, depending on where you live and whether it is an American or foreign adoption.

24. *How expensive is it to adopt a child?*

Adoptions arranged through county or state welfare agencies have very few fees. Adoptions arranged through private religious or non-religious licensed agencies cost between $1,500 and $6,000. Some agencies have a sliding fee schedule based on family income. Private, non-licensed adoptions arranged through an intermediary attorney or physician may cost as much as $25,000.

25. *Are foreign adoptions more expensive?*

Yes, they usually are. In addition to normal adoption fees, someone must pick up the baby or you must pay for someone to escort the baby to this country. There also may be immigration fees. In addition, some couples have an attorney represent them to make sure legal procedures are performed properly, which also adds to the cost.

26. *Do many couples decide not to adopt?*

Many couples decide they will have their own baby or not have a child at all. This is a valid alternative and should not be overlooked. It may take some thought and effort to get to that point, but it can be satisfying for couples to make that decision, then go on with their lives.

We live in a world today where there are opportunities to have contact with children through Big Brother and Big Sister programs, community programs and recreational activities. Many childless couples find these contacts, along with special relationships with children of family members and friends, to be satisfying, child-centered experiences.

Glossary

Abortion—Premature loss of a pregnancy.

Abruptio placenta—Premature separation of a normally *attached* placenta.

Acquired Immune Deficiency Syndrome (AIDS)—Viral disease that affects the immune system and prevents the body from fighting off common illnesses. It is prevalent among homosexuals but can be transmitted by blood transfusions and intimate contact with body fluids, such as saliva and semen. A few cases have been reported of women getting the disease from donor semen inseminations; this is one reason for the decrease in use of fresh semen in donor inseminations.

Adenoma—Growth or tumor larger than 1cm.

Adenomyosis—Condition in which endometrial tissue grows into the uterine muscle wall; it may cause severe menstrual cramps. It is often called *internal endometriosis.*

Adhesions—Fibrous structure by which parts of the body abnormally adhere to each other. Adhesions may form after pelvic infections, as a result of endometriosis and after abdominal and pelvic surgery.

Adrenal gland—Small gland situated above each kidney; it is responsible for controlling sugar and salt metabolism. Abnormalities of hormone secretion from the adrenal may cause infertility by interfering with FSH and LH.

Adrenocorticoptropic hormone (ACTH)—Hormone produced by the pituitary gland; it regulates hormonal production of the adrenal gland.

Agglutination—Clumping together of a particular substance. Sperm agglutination occurs if there is a head-to-head or tail-to-tail clumping of sperm, which may indicate an infection in the prostrate gland.

Allergic—Hypersensitivity to a specific substance, such as cervical mucus that immobilizes sperm.

Amenorrhea—Absence or abnormal cessation of a woman's periods.

Amenorrhea-galactorrhea—Condition in which periods cease (amenorrhea) and a milklike substance is secreted from the breasts (galactorrhea). It may be caused by a pituitary-gland tumor, various medications or some serious illnesses.

Androgenic—Producing masculine characteristics.

Androgens—Male sex hormone or synthetic substance that can give rise to masculine characteristics.

Andrologist—Physician who specializes in study of male hormones, sperm production and sperm transport.

Anesthesia—Loss of feeling or sensation. General anesthesia refers to total loss of consciousness or "being put to sleep." Local or regional anesthesia refers to certain region of body being anesthetized, such as in a spinal anesthetic or local anesthetic.

Anosmia—Loss of sense of smell.

Anovulation—Suspension or cessation of ovulation.

Antibiotic—Chemical substance that destroys or inhibits bacterial growth to combat infections.

Antibody—Protein substance produced by the body in response to antigenic stimulation.

Antigen—Protein or protein complex that stimulates the body's immune system to produce antibodies.

Artificial insemination—Artificially placing semen or sperm from a man into the vagina, cervical canal or intrauterine cavity in a woman to achieve pregnancy.

Artificial insemination, donor (AID)—Artificial insemination in which semen or sperm is from someone other than the husband.

Artificial insemination, husband (AIH)—Artificial insemination in which semen or sperm is from the husband.

Asherman's Syndrome—Scar tissue forms in the uterine cavity, which prevents normal uterine lining from developing. Most commonly seen after a D&C following an infected abortion or miscarriage.

Autoimmune disease—Disease that is brought on because the body destroys its own tissue.

Bartholin duct cyst—Cyst formed by plugging of Bartholin gland duct, resulting in a swollen, tender cyst in the labia majora that may have to be drained surgically.

Bartholin gland—Gland located on each side of the vaginal opening in the vulva that contributes to lubrication during intercourse. Also called *vulvo-vaginal gland*.

Basal body temperature graph (BBT)—Graph to record a woman's at-rest (basal) temperature. If she is ovulating, there usually is a slight rise (0.6 degree) in her temperature that occurs after ovulation and remains elevated until her next period.

Basal temperature—Temperature of the body when it is at total rest.

Biopsy—Removal and examination of tissue from the body to make a diagnosis.

Blighted ovum—Fertilized egg that fails to develop into a fetus following implantation in uterus. Resulting pregnancy usually results in a spontaneous miscarriage because amniotic sac is filled with fluid.

Bromocryptine—Generic name for drug Parlodel.

Cauterization—Burning or application of caustic substance to destroy tissue. It is commonly used on the cervix to treat chronic cervicitis or the Fallopian tubes for sterilization.

Cervical canal polyps—Benign growths that begin in the endocervical canal; they may protrude through the cervical opening causing abnormal vaginal bleeding.

Cervical conization—Surgical procedure in which a cone-shaped piece of tissue is removed from the center of the cervix. This may result in a weakening of the cervix (incompetent cervix) or complete removal of mucus-producing cells so sperm cannot get into the uterus.

Cervical eversion—Condition in which mucus-producing cells that normally line the cervical canal (endocervix) grow more outwardly on the cervix (exocervix) resulting in a "raw-looking" cervix covered with cervical mucus. Cells can become infected and result in thick, non-penetrable mucus that immobilizes sperm when it enters mucus.

Cervical mucus-sperm-penetration assay—Infertility test in which sperm and cervical mucus are mixed together to determine compatibility between them.

Cervicitis—Inflammation or infection of the cervix that may cause an abnormal discharge, preventing sperm from entering the uterine cavity and Fallopian tubes.

Cervix—Neck of the uterus that produces mucus that allows sperm to enter the uterine cavity on the way to the Fallopian tube. Cervix is scraped when a Pap smear is done, and it dilates during labor.

Chancre—Primary lesion of syphilis. It appears as a small, ulcerated, non-tender sore and may be present on any of the genital organs or or in the mouth. Syphilis usually does not affect fertility but may affect the developing baby when pregnancy occurs.

Chlamydia—Sexually transmitted disease that may result in cervicitis or PID, resulting in poor cervical mucus or blocked Fallopian tubes.

Chocolate cyst—Ovarian cyst filled with old, dried blood resembling chocolate. It usually results from the bleeding of endometrial glands implanted in the ovary.

Chromosomes—Small rod-shaped structures found in all body cells; they contain genes (hereditary factors) that are passed from parent to child.

Cilia—Fine, hairlike structures that line the internal surface of the Fallopian tubes; they "sweep" the egg down the Fallopian tube toward the uterus.

Clitoris—Small, elongated erectile body in a woman that is sensitive to sexual stimulation.

Clomid—Medication to stimulate ovulation in a woman and sperm production in a man. It is the brand name for clomiphene citrate.

Clomiphene citrate—Synthetic chemical that stimulates ovulation in a woman and sperm production in a man.

Complete miscarriage—Miscarriage in which uterine contents are completely expelled.

Conception—Fertilization of egg by the sperm, which results in pregnancy. To conceive means to become pregnant.

Condom—Sheath placed on a man's erect penis before intercourse to prevent sperm from entering the vagina.

Condom therapy—Treatment used in some cases of immunologic or allergic infertility to decrease immune response of cervical mucus to sperm.

Condyloma latum—Broad, flat, warty growth cause by syphilis. These do not interfere with fertility but can be a sign of secondary syphilis, which may affect a developing fetus.

Condylomata acuminata—Viral infection that causes warts to grow in a man or woman. Warts may be found on the cervix, vagina, labia, urethra, anus, penis or scrotum. They are also called *venereal warts.*

Congenital anomalies—Birth defects. About 3% of all infants are born with birth defects that may be caused by viruses, drugs, medications and other conditions.

Conservative surgery—Term used for surgery performed on the uterus, Fallopian tubes or ovaries when the goal is to preserve childbearing by not removing organs. It is commonly done for surgery for endometriosis and PID.

Contraception—Prevention of conception or pregnancy.

Contraceptive—Anything used to prevent pregnancy.

Contraceptive jelly—Jelly that kills sperm; used in association with a diaphragm to prevent conception.

Contraceptive sponge—Small sponge that contains a spermicide; when placed in the vagina against the cervix it acts as a barrier-method of birth control.

Corpus luteum—Organ that forms in the ovary after ovulation that produces progesterone. If pregnancy occurs, the corpus luteum produces progesterone to support the implantation until the placenta takes over production of progesterone.

Corpus luteum cyst—Cyst that occasionally develops from the corpus luteum, either after ovulation or from a corpus luteum of pregnancy.

Cortisone—Hormone produced by the adrenal gland; it helps the body metabolize sugar and salt. It may be used in certain ovulation disorders if overproduction of hormones from the adrenal gland are suspected.

Cowper's gland—Pair of small glands located at the base of the penis that contribute to the seminal fluid in the ejaculate.

Cryosurgery—Surgical procedure that utilizes freezing to remove abnormal tissue. It is often used to treat abnormal cells or excessive mucus-secreting cells on the cervix.

Cryptorchidism—Medical term for undescended testicles.

CT scan—Diagnostic X-ray procedure that uses computers to project an image on X-ray film.

Culdoscopy—Examination in which a fiberoptic endoscope (culdoscope) is placed through the vagina, into the pelvic cavity to see the uterus, tubes and ovaries.

Culture—Laboratory test used to grow certain microorganisms to determine the cause of an infectious disease. It is helpful in selecting the type of antibiotic a person needs to treat an infection.

Cyst—Sac that contains a liquid or semisolid substance. Some cysts, especially on the ovary, are related to normal ovarian function while other cysts can be a sign of an abnormal growth or tumor.

Danazol—Synthetic hormone medication that causes pseudomenopause. It is used in treatment of endometriosis to suppress growth of endometriosis glands.

Dehydryoepiandosterone sulfate (DHEAS)—Hormone secreted by the adrenal gland; if present in increased amounts it may interfere with ovulation.

Depo-provera—Injectable, long-acting progesterone used to treat endometriosis and other gynecologic conditions.

Diaphragm—Molded rubber cap used with contraceptive jelly to provide a barrier method of contraception. It is occasionally used in artificial insemination to keep sperm in contact with the cervix after insemination.

Diethystilbestrol (DES)—Synthetic female hormone used during the 1940s and '50s to treat abnormal bleeding during pregnancy and threatened miscarriages. It has been shown to cause abnormalities of the reproductive systems in children born to mothers treated with DES during pregnancy.

Dilatation and curettage (D&C)—Surgical procedure in which cervix is dilated to allow spoon-shaped instrument (curette) into the uterus to scrape uterine lining. It is used to treat and diagnose abnormal uterine bleeding and to remove remaining pregnancy tissue after a miscarriage.

Dysmenorrhea—Painful menstrual periods.

Dyspareunia—Painful intercourse.

Ectopic pregnancy—Pregnancy that implants and grows anywhere other than in the uterine cavity. They commonly occur in the Fallopian tube but may also occur on the ovary, cervix or abdominal cavity.

Ejaculate—Seminal fluid discharge at the time of an ejaculation in the male consisting of sperm and secretions from the Cowper's glands, epididymis, vas deferens, seminal vesicles and prostate.

Elective abortion—Elective termination of a pregnancy.

Embryo—Developing egg from 1 week after conception to the end of 8 weeks.

Embryo transfer—Term used to describe transfer of a fertilized egg into the uterus of a woman. It is used in in-vitro fertilization in which fertilization takes place in a test tube then fertilized egg is transferred to a woman's uterus or when an embryo is taken from one woman's uterus and transferred to another woman.

Endocrine glands—Gland that secretes hormones that have a specific effect on another organ of the body. The pituitary gland, thyroid gland, adrenal gland, testicle and ovary are all endocrine glands.

Endocrinologist—Physician who specializes in diseases of the endocrine glands.

Endometrial biopsy—Biopsy of endometrium used in infertility investigation to determine if ovulation has occurred. It is performed by removing a small piece of tissue and sending it to a pathologist for microscopic examination.

Endometrioma—Growth or cyst in the ovary consisting of endometriosis glands and dried blood. It is also called a *chocolate cyst*.

Endometriosis—Condition in which tissue resembling uterine lining occurs outside the uterus, such as on the ovaries, Fallopian tubes and pelvic ligaments. Endometriosis is often associated with infertility.

Endometritis—Inflammation or infection of endometrium.

Endometrium—Membrane that lines internal surface of the uterus. This membrane sheds when a woman has a menstrual period, and it is where a normal pregnancy implants after fertilization.

Endoscope—Instrument connected to a fiberoptic light source; used to examine the inside of the bladder, uterus or abdominal cavity. Hysteroscope, laparoscope and culdoscope are different types of endoscopes used in infertility investigations.

Epididymis—During their development, sperm enter epididymis after leaving the testicle. It is in the epididymis that sperm obtain their ability to fertilize an egg.

Epididymitis—Inflammation or infection of the epididymis.

Estrogens—Group of female hormones, secreted by ovaries, that are responsible for a woman's female characteristics, such as breast development and menstruation.

Fallopian tubes—Long, slender tubes that extend from the upper lateral angle of the uterus toward the ovaries on each side. Tubes pick up the egg after ovulation; it is the place where fertilization normally occurs.

Fertility specialist—Physician who specializes in treating individuals who have difficulty becoming pregnant.

Fertilization—Sperm uniting with the egg, which results in the start of a pregnancy.

Fibroid tumor—Growth of uterine muscle fibers, also called *myoma* or *leiomyoma*. Fibroids may interfere with a woman becoming pregnant.

Fimbria—Fingerlike projections at the end of the Fallopian tube that pick up egg at time of ovulation.

Fimbriectomy—Removal of fimbria in tubal sterilization procedure.

Follicular stimulating hormone (FSH)—Hormone secreted by the pituitary gland that causes egg to mature in the ovary and sperm to be produced in the testicle.

Frozen embryo—Freezing a fertilized egg to save for future use, such as in-vitro fertilization. Several eggs can be obtained during laparoscopy, fertilized and saved for later use so laparoscopy does not have to be repeated for each embryo transfer.

Fructose test—Test to determine if fructose is present in the semen. If fructose is not present, it indicates a blockage in the man's ductal system.

Galactorrhea—Excessive or spontaneous flow of milk from the breast. In the non-nursing state, it may be a sign of a small pituitary tumor with excessive secretion of prolactin.

Gamete—Ovum or sperm; when the two unite, it results in the beginning of an embryo.

Gardnerella—Bacteria that causes a vaginal infection characterized by a fishy odor and a light-green discharge. It may cause infertility by interfering with the pH balance of the vagina and with the production of cervical mucus.

Genes—Biologic unit on chromosomes by which hereditary characteristics are transmitted and determined.

Genital herpes—Herpes that occurs in the genital area.

Genitals—Reproductive organs of men and women.

Glucocorticoids—Group of hormones produced by the adrenal gland that controls sugar metabolism.

Gonadotropin—Substance that stimulates gonads; hormones FSH and LH.

Gonadotropin releasing hormone (GNRH)—Hormone produced by hypothalmus that stimulates pituitary gland to secrete FSH and LH.

Gonnorhea—Sexually transmitted disease that may cause cervicitis (inflammation of the cervix) and progress to an infection of the Fallopian tubes and ovaries, resulting in infertility.

Gynecologist—Physician who treats conditions and diseases of the genital tract in women.

Habitual miscarriage—Three or more consecutive miscarriages.

Hamster-egg-penetration assay—Laboratory test to determine the ability of sperm to fertilize an egg. Test is performed by mixing sperm from the husband with several eggs from a superovulated hamster. Eggs and sperm are incubated, and eggs are later checked for sperm penetration.

Hemophilus vaginalis—Bacteria that may cause a vaginal infection; another name for gardnerella.

Herpes—Viral infection that causes small ulcerations on the mucous membranes of the body. Cold sores and cankers are caused by herpes virus. Herpes may be contracted through sexual contact and is a sexually transmitted disease. There is no cure. Disease may be characterized by intermittent recurrences without new exposure; it has no effect on fertility.

Hormone—Chemical secreted by endocrine glands that affects other organs. GNRH, LH, FSH, progesterone, estrogen and testosterone are hormones related to fertility.

Hostile cervical mucus—Cervical mucus in which sperm are unable to survive.

Huhner's test—Another name for post-coital test.

Human chronic gonadotropin (HCG)—Hormone secreted by the placenta; it is the basis for all pregnancy tests. HCG is also used in concentrated forms to induce ovulation.

Hydrocele—Collection of fluid around the testicles that may affect testicular temperature, with subsequent effect on sperm production. A hydrocele must be found on both testicles to affect sperm count.

Hymen—Membranous fold of vaginal tissue that partially covers the vaginal opening. It occasionally remains intact or is very tight, requiring surgery before intercourse can occur.

Hyperplasia—Abnormal increase in the number of cells composing a tissue or organ, such as in adrenal or endometrial hyperplasia.

Hypospadias—Congenital birth defect of the penis in which the urethral opening occurs on the underside of the penis rather than at the end.

Hypothalmus—Area in the brain that secretes GNRH, which stimulates the pituitary gland to secrete hormones.

Hysterectomy—Surgical removal of the uterus.

Hysterogram—Test in which radiopaque dye (dye that can be seen on X-ray) is injected through the cervix, into the uterus to outline the uterine cavity and to determine if the Fallopian tubes are open. Also called *hysterosalpingogram* or *HSG*.

Hysteroscopy—Procedure used to look directly inside the uterine cavity by using a fiberoptic endoscope (hysteroscope) to see if abnormalities are present. It is performed by placing the hysteroscope through the vagina and cervix, directly into the uterine cavity.

Immune—To be protected against a particular disease.

Implantation—Process in which fertilized egg embeds in the uterine lining to continue development.

Impotence—A man's inability to have an erection and/or to ejaculate.

In-vitro fertilization—Procedure in which pregnancy is achieved by combining the egg and sperm outside the body, then later reinserting the fertilized egg into the uterus, where it will hopefully implant and continue to grow. Another name is "test-tube baby."

In-vivo fertilization—Artificial method of fertilization that occurs in the body in contrast to in-vitro fertilization, which is fertilization outside the body.

Incompetent cervix—Internal opening of the cervix is weakened and unable to hold a pregnancy to term.

Incomplete miscarriage—Tissue remains in the uterus after a miscarriage. It requires a D&C or suction curettage to remove it all.

Incubation—Time it takes to show symptoms of a disease after exposure to disease-causing organism.

Infertility—Inability to become pregnant after trying for a period of 1 year.

Infertility work-up—Investigation of an infertile couple to discover the cause for infertility.

Insemination—Deposit of seminal fluid in the vagina.

Intercourse—Sexual union in which the erect penis of a man is inserted into the vagina of a woman.

Intrauterine device (IUD)—Device inserted into the uterine cavity to prevent pregnancy.

Intrauterine insemination—Artificial method of conception in which semen or sperm is placed directly into the uterine cavity. It is used in an attempt to bypass hostile cervical mucus or other cervical factors causing infertility.

Kallman's Syndrome—Condition in which the hypothalmus in a man fails to secrete the proper amount of GNRH, which results in improper stimulation of FSH and LH and poor sperm production.

Karyotype—Chromosomal makeup of a cell. Normal chromosomal makeup is 46 XY in a man and 46 XX in a woman.

Klinefelter's Syndrome—Chromosomal abnormality in a man in which his sex chromosome is XXY instead of XY. Condition is characterized by enlarged breasts, decreased gonadotropin secretion and scarring of the seminiferous tubules of the testicles, resulting in an absence of sperm production and sterility.

Labia majora—Hairy outer folds on each side of the vagina that contain the sebaceous and sweat glands; often called the *outer lips*.

Labia minora—Two thin skin folds inside the labia majora; often called the *inner lips*.

Laparoscopy—Fiberoptic endoscope, called a *laparoscope*, is placed through the umbilicus (navel) to look directly at the uterus, Fallopian tubes and ovaries. Procedure has many uses—diagnosing pelvic pain and endometriosis, determining if Fallopian tubes are open and performing tubal sterilization.

Leydig cells—Cells in the testicle responsible for the secretion of testosterone.

Ligation—To tie off a blood vessel or tube, such as varicocele ligation or tubal ligation.

Liquefaction—Process in which semen changes from a thick, gummy state to a liquid state after ejaculation.

Luteal phase defect—Condition in which there is an inadequate production of progesterone by the corpus luteum of the ovary following ovulation. This results in a short interval between ovulation and the onset of the next menstrual period. Luteal phase defect may be a factor in infertility or cause an early miscarriage.

Luteininzing hormone (LH)—Hormone secreted by the pituitary gland that triggers ovulation. Usually a surge of LH occurs between 12 and 36 hours before ovulation; its determination is the basis for various ovulation-predictor tests.

Maturation—Process of becoming mature.

Maturation arrest—Developmental abnormality of the testicles in which sperm do not fully develop and are incapable of fertilizing an egg.

Menses—Monthly flow of blood from a woman's uterus.

Menstruation—Uterine bleeding that normally occurs at 4-week intervals in a woman. It is commonly called a *period*.

Microadenoma—Very small growth or tumor, usually less than 1cm.

Microsurgery—Surgery performed using an operating microscope or magnifying glasses to magnify tissue being operated on. Commonly used in tubal- and vasectomy-reversal surgery to give a better view of tissue.

Mineralcorticoids—Group of hormones secreted by the adrenal gland that regulates the sodium and potassium secretion.

Miscarriage—Loss of a pregnancy before the 20th week. It is the common term for a spontaneous abortion.

Missionary position—Position during intercourse in which the man is on top and the woman is on the bottom, on her back.

Mittleschmerz—Lower abdominal pain experienced by some women at the time of ovulation. Pain is usually caused by a small amount of blood or fluid discharged from the ovary when the egg is expelled, causing irritation to the pelvic peritoneum.

Morphology—Sperm characteristic present in a semen analysis that refers to normal-looking sperm.

Morula—Early stage of development of the fertilized egg in which it is just a large clump of cells. Stage just before the formation of the embryo.

Motility—Sperm movement.

Mumps orchitis—Swelling of testicles caused by mumps infection in an adult man, which may result in sterility.

Mycoplasma—Microorganism that can cause infertility by causing cervicitis or PID.

Myoma—Benign tumor of uterine muscle fibers. Commonly called a *fibroid tumor*.

Myomectomy—Surgical procedure in which myomas are removed from the uterus.

Obstetrician—Physician who cares for a pregnant woman and delivers her baby.

Oophorectomy—Surgical removal of ovaries. Unilateral oophorectomy means removing one ovary; bilateral oophorectomy means removing both ovaries.

Oral contraceptive—Birth-control pill.

Orgasm—Peak of sexual excitement or sexual climax.

Ovarian cyst—Saclike structure in the ovary that causes enlargement of the ovary. An ovarian cyst may have many causes, some related to the normal function of the ovary (follicular and corpus luteum cysts) and others caused by benign or malignant tumors of the ovary.

Ovarian failure—Ovary stops producing eggs and ovarian hormones. Menopause, which usually occurs around age 50, is caused by ovarian failure. Occasionally, ovaries stop functioning at a much earlier age; this is called *premature ovarian failure*.

Ovarian wedge resection—Surgical procedure performed on ovaries in which 25 to 40% of each ovary is removed. The purpose is to decrease hormone production of the ovaries so they will resume normal ovulation. It is usually performed in cases of polycystic ovarian disease that does not respond to clomiphene citrate.

Ovary—Female sexual gland in which eggs are formed and estrogen produced.

Ovulation—Discharge of a ripe, unfertilized egg from the ovary.

Ovulation-predictor tests—Home test done on a woman's urine to measure the surge in LH, which peaks 12 to 36 hours *before* ovulation.

Ovum—Female reproductive cell or egg.

PID—See *pelvic inflammatory disease*.

Pap smear—Test done in which cells are removed from the cervix and placed on a slide for microscopic examination. Test is used to diagnose cancerous or precancerous conditions of the cervix. Named after the Greek physician, George N. Papanicolaou.

Paracervical block—Regional anesthesia; anesthetic is injected into the cervix to numb the paracervical nerves. It is used to lessen pain and cramps in certain procedures, such as a D&C and hysterograms. It can also be used during labor to control labor pains.

Parlodel—Brand name for bromocryptine, which decreases secretion of prolactin. Drug is used to prevent engorgement of the breasts in a non-nursing mother following delivery of a baby and is also used in some cases of infertility associated with an elevated prolactin level.

Pathologist—Physician trained in diagnosing cellular structure of disease. A pathologist reads Pap smears and biopsies, and examines tissue after removal during surgery.

Pelvic exam—Examination performed by a physician in which he examines a woman's reproductive tract and performs a Pap smear.

Pelvic inflammatory disease (PID)—Infection of the uterus, Fallopian tubes and ovaries that may be caused by one of many different bacteria, such as gonorrhea or chlamydia. It may result in permanent blockage and scarring of Fallopian tubes, which results in sterility.

Penis—Male reproductive organ that is made up of circular masses of spongy tissue covered with skin. It is also the organ used for urination.

Pergonal—Powerful ovulation-inducing drug made of FSH and LH; it is used to treat resistant cases of anovulation that do not respond to other measures. Drug may result in multiple eggs being released and fertilized at the same time, causing the birth of five, six and even seven babies at once.

Phlebitis—Inflammation of a vein. Thrombophlebitis means "clot in a vein."

Pituitary adenoma or microadenoma—Small tumor or growth of the pituitary gland that may cause increased secretion of a pituitary gland hormone. If it involves prolactin-secreting cells, it may cause amenorrhea-galactorrhea, with resulting infertility.

Pituitary gland—Small gland located between and behind the eyes that secretes hormones to control many important glands in the body, such as the adrenal gland, thyroid gland, ovaries and testicles. Small growths may occur in the pituitary that cause an increase in prolactin, resulting in amenorrhea, irregular menstrual periods and infertility.

Placenta—Blood-rich organ during pregnancy that serves as the communication link between the mother and her developing fetus. It supplies oxygen and nourishing substances to the fetus and produces progesterone to help maintain a developing pregnancy. Also called the *afterbirth*.

Polycystic ovarian disease—Condition characterized by multiple, small, follicular cysts of the ovaries, irregular or absence of menses, elevated androgenic hormones, abnormal hair growth and infertility. Also called *Stein-Leventhal Syndrome*.

Polyp—Growth arising from the mucous membrane of a body cavity. The most common types related to the female-reproductive tract are polyps from the endometrium and cervix which may cause obstruction of sperm penetration or interfere with implantation of the fertilized egg.

Post-coital test—Basic infertility test. A pelvic exam is performed on a woman after she has intercourse with her husband. Cervical mucus is evaluated for clearness, quantity and to see if active, motile sperm are present.

Pregnancy—Condition of having a developing embryo or fetus in the body resulting from the union of an ovum and sperm.

Premature delivery—Delivery of a baby between the 20th and 36th weeks of pregnancy.

Primary infertility—Infertility in a couple who has never conceived.

Progesterone—Hormone produced by the corpus luteum of the ovary that prepares the uterine lining for implantation. Progesterone also supports implantation during the pregnancy and is produced in large quantities by the placenta.

Prolactin—Hormone secreted by the pituitary gland that is responsible for lactation following delivery. It also may be produced by tumors of the pituitary gland that result in inhibition of ovulation and infertility.

Prostate gland—Gland in a man that surrounds the neck of the bladder and contributes fluid to the ejaculate. It is suspectible to infection, which may be a cause of male infertility.

Prostatitis—Inflammation or infection of the prostate gland.

Pseudomenopause—Condition created when danazol is used to treat endometriosis. It causes symptoms similar to menopause—amenorrhea with possible hot flashes and flushes, vaginal dryness and breast atrophy.

Pseudopregnancy—Condition created when oral contraceptives are used to treat endometriosis. It causes symptoms similar to pregnancy—amenorrhea, weight gain, nausea and bloating.

Puberty—Age at which reproductive organs become functionally operative and secondary sex characteristics begin to develop.

Purulent cervicitis—Inflamed, pus-filled cervix that can be caused by one of several organisms such as gonorrhea, chlamydia and mycoplasma. Disease affects fertility by causing very thick mucus that sperm cannot penetrate.

Radiologist—Doctor who reads X-rays.

Reproductive endocrinologist—Endocrinologist who specializes in hormones of reproduction and infertility.

Rete testis—Network of fine tubules that sperm enter after leaving the seminiferous tubules on their way into the epididymis.

Retrograde ejaculation—At ejaculation, sperm goes into the bladder rather than out the penis. The condition results in infertility because sperm do not enter the vagina or cervix.

Rubin test—Infertility test in which carbon dioxide gas in injected through the cervix, into the uterus to see if tubes are open.

Salpingectomy—Surgical removal of the Fallopian tube. It is a unilateral salpingectomy if one tube is removed and bilateral salpingectomy if both tubes are removed.

Salpingitis—Infection or inflammation of the Fallopian tubes.

Salpingoophorectomy—Surgical removal of Fallopian tubes and ovaries.

Salpingoplasty—Surgical repair of the Fallopian tube.

Scrotum—Pouch located between the legs in the male that contains the testicles and their accessory organs.

Secondary infertility—Infertility in a couple who has previously conceived.

Semen analysis—Primary test for male infertility that checks sperm count, and motility, morphology and viability of sperm. It also analyzes important semen qualities, such as its volume, thickness and alkalinity.

Semen—Total content of the male ejaculate; seminal fluid and sperm.

Seminal fluid—Liquid portion of semen or ejaculate produced by the prostate, Cowper's and seminal-vesicle glands. Part of semen without sperm.

Seminal vasography—Radiographic fertility test in which a radiopaque dye is injected into the vas deferens to see if blockage is present.

Seminal vesicles—Small saclike organ attached to the vas deferens near the urinary bladder that supplies some fluid in the ejaculate.

Seminiferous tubules—Minute folded ducts that produce sperm and make up most of the substance of the testicles.

Septum—Dividing wall within an organ. Condition may occur in the uterus and be a cause of infertility or premature delivery.

Serophene—Trade name of drug clomiphene citrate.

Sertoli-cell-only Syndrome—Congenital defect of the testicles diagnosed by testicular biopsy in which there is complete absence of sperm-producing cells, resulting in sterility.

Serum progesterone—Blood test to determine the level of progesterone in a woman's blood. Serum progesterone is elevated after ovulation occurs and is one of the tests used to document ovulation.

Skene's glands—Two small glands located near the urethral opening in a woman that may become infected and cause a vaginal discharge.

Sperm—Male reproductive cell.

Sperm bank—Laboratory where sperm are frozen and saved for later use.

Sperm count—Number of sperm found in a semen specimen.

Sperm washings—Procedure in which semen and sperm are treated with a protein solution to try to improve sperm's fertilization capabilities.

Spermatic vein ligation—Surgical procedure to treat a varicocele.

Spinnbarkeit—Elasticity or stretchiness of cervical mucus.

Split ejaculate—Semen specimen collected in two portions—the first part of the ejaculate is collected in one container and the second part in another. Purpose is to use the part with the best sperm count and motility when performing artificial insemination.

Spontaneous abortion—Loss of a pregnancy before the 20th week.

Stein-Leventhal Syndrome—See *Polycystic ovarian disease.*

Sterility—Inability to produce offspring under any circumstances; permanent infertility.

Stress pattern—Semen analysis results in which many sperm have tapered heads and poor motility; often occur in a man with a varicocele.

Stroma—Supporting tissue around endometrial glands.

Suction curettage—Removing the uterine lining using a vacuum suction machine. Procedure is used to empty the uterus during an elective termination of pregnancy (abortion) or after an incomplete miscarriage.

Surrogate mother—Substitute mother who carries a pregnancy to term for a couple who is infertile.

Swim-up technique—Type of sperm treatment in which sperm are suspended in a protein solution and allowed to swim up to the top of the solution. Active sperm that make it to the top of the solution are then concentrated and used in artificial insemination.

Syphilis—Sexually transmitted disease that enters the body through a non-tender sore. With time, the disease can spread to many other parts of the body if left untreated. Disease does not interfere with fertility but can affect a developing fetus if the disease is active during pregnancy.

T-mycoplasma—Microorganism, now called *ureaplasma urealyticum,* that can cause cervicitis and PID in a woman and urethritis and prostatitis in a man.

Teratogen—Substance that causes defects in a developing fetus.

Test-tube baby—Common name for in-vitro fertilization. Fertilization occurs outside the woman's body, in a laboratory dish or test tube.

Testicles—Male gonad situated in the scrotum that produces spermatozoa and testosterone.

Testicular biopsy—Removal of a small piece of tissue from the testicle to examine under a microscope to help evaluate the cause of male infertility.

Testicular torsion—Condition in which testicles twist on their supporting ligaments and cut off the blood supply, resulting in acute swelling and possible decay of the testicle.

Testosterone—Hormone produced by the testicle; it is responsible for development and growth of a man's sexual characteristics.

Testosterone rebound—Hormonal treatment used in some infertile men to try to improve their sperm count.

Thyroid gland—Large gland situated in front of and on either side of the trachea that secretes thyroxin, which controls metabolism.

Thyrotropic stimulating hormone (TSH)—Hormone produced by the pituitary gland that controls the thyroid gland.

Trichomonas—Single-cell organism that may cause a vaginal infection characterized by an odorous, light-green discharge.

Tubal anastamosis—Surgical procedure in which the Fallopian tubes are reconnected after a previous sterilization procedure.

Tubal ligation—Surgical procedure in which Fallopian tubes are tied, cut, burned or clipped for permanent sterilization.

Tubal pregnancy—Pregnancy that implants in the Fallopian tubes.

Tuboplasty—Surgical repair of the Fallopian tubes.

Turner's Syndrome—Woman with an XO sex-chromosome pattern characterized by short stature, webbed neck, increased carrying angle of the elbow and lack of sexual development. There are no functional ovaries, and the woman is sterile.

Ultrasound machine—Image-producing machine that uses sound waves to project an image on a monitor.

Undescended testicles—Testicles that fail to descend into the scrotum during fetal development; it may result in sterility and a predisposition to malignancy.

Unexplained infertility—Infertility for which no known cause is found.

Ureaplasma—Microorganism that can cause infertility by causing cervicitis or PID. Also causes non-specific urethritis (NSU) in men.

Urethra—Membranous canal that carries urine from the bladder to the exterior of the body. In a man, the urethra also carries the seminal fluid during ejaculation.

Urethral stricture—Narrowing of the urethra often caused by gonorrhea, which may interfere with the flow of urine.

Urethritis—Infection or inflammation of the urethra.

Urologist—Physician who specializes in disorders of the urinary system in men and women. He also specializes in disorders of the male reproductive system.

Uterine perforation—Hole made through the uterus at the time of a D&C or elective abortion that may result in excessive bleeding requiring major surgery to correct the condition.

Uterine polyp—Growth on the uterine lining that may cause abnormal uterine bleeding and interfere with implantation of a fertilized egg. Also called *endometrial polyp.*

Uterus—Hollow muscular organ in a woman that is the place of nourishment for an embryo and fetus. It consists of the body, the cervix (neck) and the endometrium (lining).

Vagina—Canal in the female extending from the vulva to the cervix, which receives the penis during intercourse.

Vaginismus—Spasm of the vagina that makes it impossible for the penis to enter the vagina during intercourse.

Vaginitis—Inflammation or infection of the vagina caused by one of several different organisms that may cause infertility by interfering with sperm survival.

Varicocele—Varicose veins around the testicle that can cause infertility by causing poor sperm development.

Vas deferens—Excretory duct of the testicles that carries the sperm from the epididymis to the urethra.

Vasectomy—Surgical procedure in which vas deferens is cut for permanent sterilization.

Venereal warts—Small warty growths caused by a virus that can occur on the genitals in either sex; warts are transmitted sexually.

Viability—Sperm characteristic present in a semen analysis that refers to the number of live sperm present.

Viscosity—Semen quality that refers to the thickness of semen after it liquefies.

Vulva—Woman's external genital organs, including the mons pubis, labia majora and other structures between the labia.

Womb—Another term for uterus.

Yeast infection—Vaginal infection caused by a fungus that results in severe vaginal itching and a white cottage-cheese discharge. It only interferes with fertility if the infection is severe and prevents intercourse or sperm survival.

Index

GNRH 12, 13, 14, 126, 157, 208
Galactorrhea 18, 19, 158, 159, 209
Gardnerella 129, 130, 260, 273
Genetic counseling 93
Genital herpes 268
Gland, adrenal 12, 13, 15, 22, 23, 24, 25, 151, 208
Gland, Bartholin 29
Gland, Cowper's 46, 178
Gland, endocrine 12, 22, 25, 96
Gland, hypothalmus 12, 13, 14, 25, 109, 125, 157, 207, 208
Gland, periurethral 201
Gland, pituitary 12, 13, 14, 15, 16, 19, 21, 23, 25, 125, 157, 158, 159, 208, 241
Gland, prostate 45, 46, 136, 178, 201, 203, 204, 205, 206, 272
Gland, Skene's 29
Gland, thyroid 12, 13, 14, 15, 20, 21, 25, 96, 151, 207, 215
Gland, vulvovaginal 29
Glucocorticoids 22
Gonadal dysgenesis 162
Gonadotropin-releasing hormone, see GNRH
Gonorrhea 134, 145, 202, 203, 204, 245, 260, 261, 262, 263, 265, 266
Growth hormone 15
Gynecomastia 212

H
HCG 74, 95, 153, 154, 155, 156, 212
HSG 96, 105, 108, 112, 113, 114, 115, 123, 127, 139, 250
Habitual miscarriage 90
Ham's solution 206, 224
Hamster-egg-penetration assay 193, 221, 222
Hemoglobin test 107
Hemophilus infection 260, 273, 274
Hemophilus vaginitis 273
Herpes 145, 260, 268, 269, 270, 276
Herpes zoster 268
Home pregnancy tests 75
Hormonal therapy 211
Hormone imbalance 151
Hormone production, excessive 106
Hormone, adrenocorticotropic 14
Hormone, growth 15
Hostile mucus 136
Hot flashes 162

Hot tubs 188
Huhner's test 110
Hydrocele 184, 195, 196
Hymen 29
Hymenectomy 29
Hymenotomy 29
Hyperplasia 23
Hypogonadotropic hypogandism 208
Hypostadias 202
Hypothalmus gland 12, 13, 14, 25, 109, 125, 157, 207, 208
Hypothyroidism 19, 159
Hypoxia 194
Hysterectomy 34, 35, 80, 149, 176, 258
Hysterogram 112, 127, 142, 145
Hysterosalpingogram 96, 105, 108, 112, 113, 114, 115, 123, 127, 139, 250
Hysteroscope 283
Hysteroscopy 97, 122, 123, 124, 139, 144

I
IUD 138, 139, 140, 147, 148, 240, 244, 245, 246
Idiopathic infertility 193
Imbalance, hormone 151
Immunologic infertility 216, 218, 222, 223, 224, 229, 280
Implantation bleeding 86
Impotence 66, 185, 209, 213, 214, 215, 292
Impotence, emotional 213, 214
Impotence, physical 214
In-vitro fertilization 118, 222, 225, 250, 251, 252, 266, 279, 280, 281, 282, 283, 284, 286
In-vivo fertilization 282, 283, 284
Incompetent cervix 96, 97, 99, 258, 259
Incomplete miscarriage 90
Infection, cervical 134, 135
Infection, prostate 183
Infection, yeast 129
Infertility evaluation 298
Infertility examination 104
Infertility investigation 216
Infertility tests 105
Infertility work up 104
Infertility, definition 103
Infertility, immunologic 216, 218, 222, 223, 224, 229, 280
Infertility, male factor 283
Infertility, unexplained 216, 220, 221, 224, 229, 280, 283
Insemination, artificial 44, 118, 134, 201,

ABOUT THE AUTHORS

Melvin J. Frisch, M.D., attended medical school at the University of Minnesota and graduated with an M.D. degree in 1966. After interning in California, he practiced family medicine for 5 years in Montana, where he was in private practice and also worked for the Indian Health Service. In 1972, he returned to the University of Minnesota to complete his residency in Obstetrics-Gynecology. Dr. Frisch is board certified by the American College of Obstetrics and Gynecology; today he practices in Minneapolis, where he has a special interest in infertility and tubal microsurgery. Dr. Frisch is also a Clinical Assistant Professor at the University of Minnesota Medical School, Chief of Surgery at Sinai Hospital in Minneapolis, Medical Director of the Annex Team Clinic in Robbinsdale, and on the staff at Meadowbrook Women's Clinic in St. Louis Park.

Gayle Rapoport, who also attended the University of Minnesota and is a former medical secretary, discovered she had secondary infertility. She became a patient of Dr. Frisch's and resolved her fertility problem under his care. While she was undergoing treatment, she wanted to find out more about the problem but was unable to do so because there weren't many books about infertility for someone who wasn't a medical professional. She realized there was a great need for information about fertility written for a layperson, so she and Dr. Frisch decided to collaborate in preparing and presenting this material.